T0314991

The Impossible Clinic

The Impossible Clinic

A Critical Sociology of
Evidence-Based Medicine

BY ARIANE HANEMAAYER

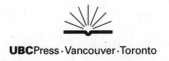

UBCPress · Vancouver · Toronto

28 27 26 25 24 23 22 21 20 19   5 4 3 2 1

Printed in Canada on FSC-certified ancient-forest-free paper (100% post-consumer recycled) that is processed chlorine- and acid-free.

Library and Archives Canada Cataloguing in Publication

Title: The impossible clinic : a critical sociology of evidence-based medicine / by Ariane Hanemaayer.
Names: Hanemaayer, Ariane, author.
Description: Includes bibliographical references.
Identifiers: Canadiana (print) 2019014114X | Canadiana (ebook) 20190141174 |
    ISBN 9780774862073 (hardcover) | ISBN 9780774862097 (PDF) |
    ISBN 9780774862103 (EPUB) | ISBN 9780774862110 (Kindle)
Subjects: LCSH: Evidence-based medicine.
Classification: LCC R723.7 .H36 2019 | DDC 616—dc23

Canadä

UBC Press gratefully acknowledges the financial support for our publishing program of the Government of Canada (through the Canada Book Fund), the Canada Council for the Arts, and the British Columbia Arts Council.

This book has been published with the help of a grant from the Canadian Federation for the Humanities and Social Sciences, through the Awards to Scholarly Publications Program, using funds provided by the Social Sciences and Humanities Research Council of Canada.

Printed and bound in Canada by Friesens
Set in Bodoni and Baskerville10Pro by Apex CoVantage, LLC
Copy editor: Joanne Richardson
Proofreader: Alison Strobel
Indexer: Stephen Ullstrom
Cover designer: David Drummond

UBC Press
The University of British Columbia
2029 West Mall
Vancouver, BC V6T 1Z2
www.ubcpress.ca

For TDPB

Contents

Preface

THE OBJECTIVES OF this book are to explain the emergence and failures of evidence-based medicine (EBM) and to offer a "soft" critique of ongoing work in biopower and governmentality studies in the sociology of health and medicine. The materials presented here respond to an opening in the literature, presented by Eric Mykhalovskiy and Lorna Weir in 2004, for a genealogy of EBM that links its emergence to clinical epidemiology. There have been many attempts within the social sciences to describe and explain EBM: What is it? Where did it come from? How do people use evidence? What role do standards play in its practice? Despite many criticisms of the weaknesses, limitations, and even contradictions surrounding the practice of EBM, there has yet to be any research that has been able to explain how it has been able to keep going despite its failures. This is due to the fact that a great deal of emphasis has been placed on the empirical, or practical, aspects of the clinic. *The Impossible Clinic* examines the force relations that organize knowledge and the effects of the institutional techniques that regulate clinical practice. In other words, it analyzes the taxonomies that make clinical perception possible and explains the domination of liberal governance that allows EBM to keep going.

I organize the book according to Foucauldian criteria, and I posit that a "dispositif" (see below) has congealed in modern Western medicine. The first four chapters engage in an empirical analysis of the emergence of EBM, clinical practice guidelines, and a database of disciplinary decisions that I constructed from the English provincial colleges of medicine across Canada. All these materials have been collected and presented in such a way as to persuade you, the reader, of my position: EBM is an impossible project. This, I hope, will lead to advances in the sociology of medicine, the sociology of health, and governmentality studies, all of which have been concerned with describing the tactics of self-governance in liberal programs of conduct. Much of that literature, even in health and medicine, has sought to define individual subjectivity as regulated through the self-recognition of the ethical duty to improve one's capacities to judge, to become better at making decisions to improve oneself, one's health, and one's capacity for making these decisions. I believe, for reasons that I spell out through both my empirical research and theoretical engagement with Foucault's method and analytic, that the convergence of forces among liberal governance and professional strategies merits alternate conceptualizations of how subjects externalize their judgments through professional regulation. Taking this tack seriously means that I move away from a conceptualization of subjects that are, in the words of Paul Rabinow and Nikolas Rose (2006, 197), "brought to work on themselves." I term this effect "deresponsibilization," a concept that has yet to be used in the sociology of medicine literature. This effect is antithetical to EBM's goal to responsibilize self-learners to keep up with and to appraise evidence, and thus signifies its failure as a liberal program of conduct.

I understand that not all readers read from cover to cover, so I begin each chapter with a brief summary of the chains of reasoning necessary to understand it. The chapters are ordered to explain how the techniques used by EBM to intervene in the clinic came to congeal within a dispositif, a set-up, in the words of Paul Veyne, through an assemblage of regulatory policies, professional knowledge in the form of clinical practice guidelines (CPGs), and disciplinary and normalizing strategies of power. These relations have been institutionalized across a variety of sites of practice, and I explain how they have converged among medical education, clinical sciences, governmental agencies, and the professional corporations of Canada's medical colleges. The deployment of CPGs as categories of knowledge that ought to organize clinical activity is, in effect, impossible as they produce effects that fail to meet the objectives of EBM. In *Discipline and Punish,* Foucault analyzes the prison as a policy program that coordinates punishment, and he argues that the panoptic prison and the disciplinary society is impossible, yet it persists. Drawing on a genealogical method, I am able to explain how EBM, through its use of CPGs, is able to persist even though it is antithetical to its own goals. By examining the links between disciplinary strategies in medical regulation and the knowledge that organizes clinical activity (CPGs), I find the same impossibility Foucault outlines in his analysis of the prison.

In writing this book I hope for two outcomes. First, I want to make Foucault relevant to a sociology of medicine by proposing that we ask genealogical questions about medical knowledge and strategies in addition to those concerning whether physicians actually use evidence in practice and/or how they interpret evidence – questions that have been the predominant focus of the sociology of medicine and EBM (and which may not fully capture the institutionalized dynamics of power and knowledge). Second, I want to update Foucault's archaeology of medical practice with genealogical research. I'm hoping that my application of his method to a sociology of medicine will open up his corpus to new synthetic work and show how Foucault remains helpful for explaining the relationships between medical knowledge, liberal governance, and biopower today, with an eye towards professional regulation as a key to understanding the relationships between these domains.

As with any project, in this one I had to make sociological judgments that left out many important aspects of the history (albeit recent) of EBM. I chose a careful path among the various solutions offered regarding the problems of clinical practice associated with clinical judgment. There are likely to be recognizable omissions or sections that may not have received the dedicated development they deserve. I can only justify these by recourse to a "through-line" that had to govern many of my decisions about what could be admitted to a book of this nature. I decided to focus on explaining the failures that result from the convergence of EBM, CPGs, and medical regulation; I leave the analysis of other unsuccessful attempts to solve the problems of clinical judgment to my next project, on which I am currently working. Many lines of investigation had to be sacrificed to future research, including those relations of discourse and strategies that now find themselves in public health. I am beginning to "reserialize" alternate approaches to the management of health care in various domains by showing how their dominant programs can be traced to the problematization of clinical judgment, which is where *The Impossible Clinic* begins.

As with all academic endeavours, my ability to complete this project is due to the debts that I have accrued. Many colleagues and supports, without whom and without which this project would not have come to fruition, need to be thanked. Zohreh BayatRizi, Robyn Braun, Tim Caulfield, Brendan Leier, Tara Milbrandt, Eric Mykhalovskiy, and Emma Whelan all provided substantive direction and feedback during various stages of the project. I would also like to thank Ronjon Paul Datta, whose many insights into Foucault have challenged and nurtured my own interests, with special thanks for his suggestion for the title of this book.

This work was well funded by the Killam Trust and Dalhousie University, two institutions that supported the majority of my archival research. Also, about a third of this research was completed during my doctoral work, which was funded by a Social Sciences and Humanities Research Council of Canada Doctoral Scholarship. The Department of Sociology at the University of Alberta also provided a research grant to carry out the majority of the archival research that appears in Chapter 2.

I also owe a great deal of thanks to many of the archivists who helped me along the way. The success of this project is due largely to their careful help and knowledge of the materials in their respective archives: Anne McKeage at McMaster; Peter Smith at the Royal College of Physicians and Surgeons of Canada; the archivists at the Archives of Ontario, the National Archives of the United

Kingdom, and Library and Archives Canada; and colleague Braydon O'Neill at the Centre for Evidence-Based Medicine at University of Oxford.

I would also like to thank various audiences, colleagues, and friends who listened to me work through these ideas or who offered feedback during various stages of construction: the members of the Technoscience and Regulation Research Unit at Dalhousie, the participants at the Making Standards Workshop, the Science and Technology Studies Reading Group led by Dani Inkpen, Tyler Brunet, Laura Eramian, Janice Graham, Jean-Sébastien Guy, Matthew Herder, Christina Holmes, Peter Mallory, Fiona MacDonald, Liz and Blair McLeod, and Carlos Mariscal. I'd also like to thank Darcy Cullen, my editor at UBC Press, and the anonymous peer reviewers for their careful reading and constructive feedback, from which this book has truly benefitted.

Finally, no project would be possible without the love and support of my family, John, Glenda, and Kiara, who helped me keep it all together just enough to tackle writing this book within such an ambitious timeline.

Abbreviations

AO	Archives of Ontario
CE&B	Department of Clinical Epidemiology and Biostatistics at McMaster University
CMA	Canadian Medical Association
CME	Continuing medical education
CMPA	Canadian Medical Protective Agency
CPGs	Clinical practice guidelines, also called "best practice guidelines"
CPSA	College of Physicians and Surgeons of Alberta
CPSBC	College of Physicians and Surgeons of British Columbia
CPSM	College of Physicians and Surgeons of Manitoba
CPSNB	College of Physicians and Surgeons of New Brunswick
CPSNL	College of Physicians and Surgeons of Newfoundland
CPSNS	College of Physicians and Surgeons of Nova Scotia
CPSO	College of Physicians and Surgeons of Ontario
CPSPEI	College of Physicians and Surgeons of Prince Edward Island
CPSS	College of Physicians and Surgeons of Saskatchewan
EBM	Evidence-based medicine
HCC	Health Council of Canada
JAMA	*Journal of the American Medical Association*
NA	National Archives of the United Kingdom
RCPSC	Royal College of Physicians and Surgeons of Canada
RCT	Randomized controlled trial

The Impossible Clinic

Introduction

ACCORDING TO THE *British Medical Journal,* administering soapy enemas to women during labour was a common medical practice up until the 1970s (BMJ Publishing 2014). Women were frequently subjected to this procedure on the basis that it was good for the mother and baby: mothers would not have to worry about "leakage" from their "back passage" during childbirth, which could be, according to conventional wisdom, embarrassing for them. The additional benefit, medical professionals thought, was that during delivery newborns could be protected from the slight chance of coming into contact with harmful bacteria contained in the excreted stool. While we might be suspicious that any potential embarrassment for the women could be considered barely medical in nature, the health of the baby was a primary concern: Who wouldn't support the idea that new babies are vulnerable and should be protected from health hazards early on to ensure their lives are off to the best possible start? The procedures were, as one might imagine, quite uncomfortable and even painful for women, especially when administered during an already taxing experience. But, even if she wanted to, how could a woman refuse what she was told would be "good for the baby"? On what solid basis could anyone question this medical procedure?

Ultimately, scientific study alleviated any potential concerns of mothers-to-be. Reveiz, Gaitán, and Cuervo (2000, 2, emphasis

3

added) conducted a review of the literature to assess whether enemas were, in fact, beneficial:

> These studies found no significant differences in any of the outcomes assessed either for the woman or the baby. However, none of the trials assessed pain for the woman during labour and there were insufficient data to assess rare adverse outcomes. Thus *the evidence speaks against* the routine use of enemas during labour.

By testing whether enemas were actually improving the outcome of newborn-and-mother health, the researchers determined that they were not effective. They recommended that this practice, which had been administered on the basis of a commonly held belief within the medical profession, be stopped. But how did this enema-giving practice become commonplace to begin with? On what were doctors who administered enemas before this study was released basing their judgments? Further, who initiated the idea of using research to question the judgment of physicians in the first place? And, subsequently, if research could disrupt conventional practices in the clinic, could it also be used to correct and improve that "conventional wisdom" with scientific measurement? Questions of this nature can be attributed to an approach to medical practice that would come to be known as evidence-based medicine (EBM), and they were fundamental to clinical practice reforms in the last half of the twentieth century.

This book is about the conditions that led to the emergence of EBM, which is often defined as: "The conscientious, explicit, and judicious use of current best evidence in making decisions about the care of individual patients. The practice of evidence-based medicine means integrating individual clinical expertise with the best available external clinical evidence from systematic research" (Sackett et al. 1996, 71). EBM requires that physicians consult and integrate medical (i.e., scientific) knowledge into their decisions. As such, it takes place at the level of the physician's individual judgment. "Evidence" is considered to be any research regarding the use and effectiveness of therapies and medical interventions. This research primarily relies on the use of randomized controlled trials (RCTs) (systematically executed double-blind trials of the latest therapies), the results of which are then subject to tests of statistical validity, which determine the effectiveness of an intervention in a population.

The emergence of EBM in 1992 (the date this term was first coined in the medical literature) led to the restructuring of Western medicine in less than two decades. Today, the contributions of scientific evidence are heralded as revolutionary in medical practice. By using data pertaining to the effectiveness of specific therapies and drawn from large population samples, practitioners are able to make informed judgments about their individual patients. In the past, according to Guyatt and colleagues (1992), medical practice relied heavily either on a physician's "intuition" or what was considered conventional knowledge in the field at the time. EBM, however, claims to have changed the traditional practice of medicine by adding rigorous scientific tests of validity to the results produced by scientific study. These combined results can then be entered into recommendations for actual clinical practice in the form of clinical practice guidelines (CPGs), which are a set of implemented strategies for managing disease through therapy and/or treatment programs. The administration of soapy enemas to women in labour is one example of a procedure whose basis could not be proven by measures of clinical effectiveness. Although the rationale for this practice appeared to be medically relevant (i.e., avoiding harm to the baby), it was based on flawed logic that had become convention rather than on empirical science.

The medical community praised the introduction of EBM to the clinic: "EBM has been of major value to medical practice, especially with regard to screening methodologies and therapeutics" (Schechter and Perlmanan 2009, 161). The production and collection of vast amounts of data (i.e., evidence) about new and emerging technologies and therapies has shortened the lag time between medical research and innovation and clinical practice. EBM has the power and potential to keep physicians abreast of the newest and latest tried-and-proven tests, techniques, and therapies for many known diseases or conditions. Many medical journals now focus on translating the results of medical studies into recommendations for clinical practice. EBM journals seek to improve the uptake of knowledge from laboratory research to the patient's bedside. Using evidence in clinical practice ensures that clinical care is being provided according to best practices, that the most effective recommendations are being prescribed to the public, and that doctors can be certain their judgments are based on the most up-to-date knowledge.

The example of soapy enemas presented above shows that the use of evidence in clinical practice predated the coining of the term "EBM" and its clinical method. There is a substantial amount of work in the humanities and social sciences demonstrating how medical practice was informed by evidence prior to the official appearance of EBM in the medical literature. Historians have shown that scientific evidence helped reform medicine much earlier than the pronouncement of the need for EBM. For example, the pharmaceutical market and the progress of drug research were both greatly influenced and advanced by the medical sciences (Marks 1997). EBM could not be considered "new" insofar as science had become a large part of medicine since the World Wars. What the term "EBM" provided when it appeared in 1992 was a name for a specific approach that combined methods of clinical decision making with clinical sciences, which corresponded with emerging training practices. *The Impossible Clinic* traces the emergence of this way of thinking about clinical work: it examines how the medical sciences of research became linked to bedside practice. When did this convergence first appear? What programs were put in place in medical education that enabled the uptake of evidence into practice? What forms of power converge in the medical field, and what effects do they generate? And, finally, what relations allow EBM to go on despite its identified shortcomings?

Other researchers have examined various aspects of the history and effects of EBM. Jeanne Daly (2005, 235) draws on historical evidence as well as key informant interviews to argue that EBM emerged as a result of "the development of a science of clinical care." She views both clinical epidemiology and EBM as distinct fields of science, although with much cross-fertilization (236). Clinical epidemiology defined the methods used to research the effectiveness of clinical intervention, and EBM attempts to implement this knowledge in clinical practice (206). My argument takes a different tack: clinical epidemiology emerged to respond to various problems identified with clinical practice within the medical literature. As new science, it then provided a taxonomy for the organization of clinical judgment; clinical epidemiology provided the discursive conditions of possibility for the interventions of EBM in the clinic. The implementation of evidence-based CPGs allowed EBM to intervene in clinical judgments, which, as my findings show, are now coming to be regulated at a distance by provincial medical colleges in Canada.

With regard to sociological studies of EBM, Berg (1995) demonstrates that postwar medicine reconceptualized the cognitive capacities of physicians, locating their decision-making abilities in their brains. Later, building on this research, Timmermans and Berg (2003, 8) argue that EBM was a result of standardization processes: "Evidence-based medicine is part of a wider movement to generate uniformity and quality control by streamlining processes." Like me, they see EBM as an attempt to intervene at the level of individual decision making through CPGs. Overall, they see EBM as a reaction to medical authority:

With spiraling health care costs, more emancipated patients/consumers, increasing attention to medical practice variations, an information overload, and an overall critical scrutiny of the role of experts and professionals in society, the medical profession felt it had to take unprecedented action to maintain its position as exclusive safe-keeper and wielder of medical knowledge. (Timmermans and Berg 2003, 16)

My findings show that a contingency of historical events provided EBM with more than an instrumental defence of medicine's boundaries and authority. I argue that CPGs, which Timmermans and Berg understand to be the cornerstone of EBM, are antithetical to its aims: CPGs, when used to regulate, undermine medicine; they fail to increase the physician's capacity to judge because they externalize judgment through the normalizing power of regulation.[1] I explain that this is the case because liberal forms of governance utilize the failed effects of EBM to maintain dominant forms of rule that benefit liberal objectives, such as governing medicine at a distance, responsibilizing physicians for health care, and doing little to invest in health care infrastructure. While my findings agree with those of Timmermans and Berg in many respects, specifically regarding the standardizing effects of CPGs, my objectives are to show the relations of discourse and strategies of intervention that have congealed EBM within a dispositif of liberal medicine.

Despite the support for EBM from within and beyond the medical community, it also has its critics. In just over two decades since EBM first appeared, the EBM Renaissance Group published its criticism in the *British Medical Journal*. The authors argue that EBM is in crisis. The fact that now there is just too much evidence and, as a consequence, too many guidelines is among the problems they highlight. They also worry that medicine has, as a result of the proliferation of guidelines, an "overemphasis on algorithmic rules" (Greenhalgh, Howick, and Maskery 2014): following guidelines might be replacing individual expertise and decision making. They suggest that medicine needs to reinvigorate clinical expertise and training in decision making, and "reorient" doctors away from rule following. How did medicine go from using evidence to improve clinical judgment to emphasizing rule following? To answer this question, I explain the social conditions that led to the uptake of EBM and the implementation of CPGs, and the consequences thereof. I not only confirm that CPGs are being used to punish and regulate doctors but also explain how and why.

The Impossible Clinic argues that EBM has had an effect on medical regulation in Canada. Chapter 1 shows how EBM emerged from problematizing clinical judgment in the literature of medical practice, which includes addressing the following themes: the disjuncture between the laboratory and the clinic, practice variation, and medical authority. The emerging science of clinical epidemiology sought to remedy these identified problems, which I explore in Chapter 2 through a case study of the creation of McMaster University medical school, the home of the EBM Working Group and the place where these new methods emerged. Chapter 3 demonstrates how the reform of medical education required new teaching methods, such as problem-based learning, to train physicians to become lifelong learners, to stay up to date with new information, and to apply the best evidence in their practice through the critical appraisal method. I show that new training programs responsibilized a new kind of student, one who had to keep up with new information and apply it in their practice beyond graduation.

Emerging programs in continuing medical education were created to encourage physicians to use the latest evidence in their practice and thus to keep up to date. In Chapter 4, I argue that EBM served to stabilize the use of CPGs in practice – the time constraints on practising physicians made it nearly impossible to keep up with new information. Evidence-based guidelines, it was reasoned, would make it easier for physicians to apply evidence at the bedside. Physicians' responsibility to maintain their competence with the use of new information, however, would later fall under the oversight of the provincial colleges, who were charged with licensing them and maintaining professional standards, which, after EBM, meant using the best evidence in practice. I constructed a database of disciplinary decisions to show that guidelines are being used to justify sanctions for professional misconduct. The professionalization of expertise externalizes the judgment of the physician, and this is antithetical to the aims of EBM as it reduces clinical judgment to the use of guidelines over and above improved decision making. I now turn to a discussion of the theoretical and methodological rationale of this book.

Foucauldian Genealogy and the Sociology of Medicine

While it may seem both obvious and cliché to engage with Foucault in a contemporary study of the profession of medicine, my reasons for doing so are guided by an interest in the ability of Foucault's genealogical method to, in the words of William Walters (2012, 118), "[denaturalize] objects and subjects, identities and practices that might otherwise appear given to us." Genealogy offered me the critical gaze by which I could historicize the emergence of EBM not only as the triumph of a new clinical science that rescued medicine from its limitations and improved clinical care but also as a field of knowledge deployed to regulate clinical activity. I examined the various forces and debates that were "at play," to paraphrase Foucault, leading up to the first statements of EBM; by conceptualizing medicine as a contested field, a place where emerging concerns and a "will to knowledge" about clinical reasoning became the dominant conversation. Genealogy is a suitable method for my research because it allows me to pose and answer questions about the history of EBM, its various dimensions of knowledge production, and how that knowledge comes to structure and organize human activity. Foucault's analytic of power offers a terrain on which to observe the regulatory mechanisms of the profession of medicine and to explain how their ontological status in a field of discursive practices was established. It also shows how the codification of medical judgments serves as an instrument to illuminate and introduce "all the shading of individual difference" between the individual's judgment and the norm (Foucault 1979, 184). Genealogy informs my sociological analysis in the following ways: it enables me to pay attention to the contingent lines of descent that allowed CPGs to emerge, to explain that CPGs are mobilized by force relations that normalize the profession of medicine, and to explain the effects of CPGs on institutional and discursive practices. Foucault's analytic of power provides me with my methodological rationale for writing this book.

Method and Methodology

Because the history of EBM has been written by both historians and social scientists (e.g., see Daly 2005, or Cassels 2015), many of the key players have already been interviewed, and connections between those individuals who had similar instrumental and laudable interests have been mapped within networks. Many of these stories share and reinforce a dominant narrative about those individuals who sought to remedy the ailments of unscientific practice, and their successes have resulted in EBM. These works spotlight important contributions to modern medicine, but they do not seek to explain the social and political landscapes within which their voices gained traction: What were the social conditions that allowed clinical practice to change so rapidly and clinical sciences to flourish? And why, if EBM was such a success, are there ongoing concerns about the dangers of evidence-based guidelines? If EBM fixes unscientific medicine, then is there any truth to the claim that it is in crisis? *The Impossible Clinic* concludes that clinical epidemiology emerged as a response to institutionally identified problems within clinical practice. The taxonomies of clinical judgment served to found and justify new tactics for regulating medicine, inculcating educational reform at McMaster University in Ontario and (later) across Western medicine globally, and creating evidence-based CPGs, which, when deployed through disciplinary strategies aimed at professional regulation, produce effects that are antithetical to the objectives of EBM. Critical appraisal and evidence-based medicine contradict each other, yet EBM occurs because it has congealed within a dispositif. My goal in this book is to provide an *effective history* of EBM[2] – one that has yet to be portrayed in the humanities and social sciences literature.

In investigating how the institution of medicine came to educate practitioners through the use of EBM, I relied on two main sources: 1) general medical journals that have been in circulation in Canada, the United States, and the United Kingdom since the mid-twentieth century and 2) archival materials. The term "evidence-based medicine" was first coined by clinical researchers at McMaster University in Ontario, Canada. Research was carried out in the Archives of Ontario (AO), the National Archives of the United Kingdom (NA), the Royal College of Physicians and Surgeons of Canada (RCPSC) Archive, and at the McMaster University Faculty of Medicine Archives (McMaster Archives). I chose the Archives of Ontario for their policy documents, which pertain to the creation of new medical education programs in Ontario. I explored how the McMaster University medical school was created and what discursive and political influences shaped its objectives. I examined documents at the National Archives of the United Kingdom in order to understand what funding initiatives supported the international proliferation of clinical epidemiology and the creation of the Centre for Evidence-Based Medicine in 1995. The RCPSC Archives contain important documents concerning the regulation of continuing education and professional competence. The Faculty of Medicine Archives at McMaster University contain numerous documents pertaining to the history of both the clinical epidemiology program and the medical school. I examined historical documents both for the discursive rationale for the creation of the medical school program and for the political relationships between medical practitioners, university administrators, and government officials. These documents demonstrate not only how the questions in the literature were institutionalized in various training programs targeted directly at the education of clinical practitioners but also how material conditions organized the activities of medical training. I also collected archival materials that were published by the English-speaking provincial colleges of physicians and surgeons across Canada. These materials include medical acts, college-endorsed policies, and CPGs as well as the disciplinary decisions from 2010 to 2016. I examined these statements for evidence of the use of CPGs as a measure of professional misconduct across Canada.

This method allowed me to analyze clinical epidemiology, and later EBM, from within an archive of medical statements about an emergent mode of reasoning. Foucault (1972, 57) defines the archive as "the set of discourses actually pronounced ... as a set that continues to function, to be transformed through history, and to provide the possibility of appearing in other discourses." The archive holds various discourses, or collections of statements, about social phenomena that are not discipline- or context-dependent. The archive is understood to be a repository of statements that deem what is and what is not true of various human activities. Within each "layer" of the archive, certain systems of thought become dominant. Archival work "aims to explain the regularities of these archival statements" as the archive contains "the conditions of possibility for the practical know-how of subjects engaged in knowing" (Datta 2007, 278–79). "Know-how" includes the activities of doctors within the clinic. Genealogical analysis aims to show the "structuring of thought and life" by introducing the role of knowledge in organizing power relations (286). Statements are understood as "events" within a discourse (Foucault 1972, 4), and documents are understood as "monuments" that have enduring historical significance (7). Documents are created to represent and say something authoritative about a phenomenon. I analyzed archival documents for their veridical and juridical statements about social objects/practices, and how these related to the organization of human activity in the clinic.[3]

Foucauldian genealogy developed from an engagement with the historical and theoretical work of Friedrich Nietzsche. Foucault approached the study of history as a stratification of various systems of thought that aim to produce truth statements about the "human" as an object of scientific discourse. Carrying out such research involves investigating the "lines of descent" for particular institutions, focusing on how they came to be as they are, even when they seem "complete" today (Walters 2012, 117). By understanding that clinical judgments are conceived as practices that can be learned and ameliorated, my objective is to grasp the conditions that make particular ways of judging, at particular points in time, acceptable, desirable, and viable. To paraphrase Foucault (2003, 253), the interconnection between the rules imposed on medical judgments and the reasons given for using scientific evidence can be visualized in such institutional programs as medical education. To analyze the practice of clinical judgment under EBM is to analyze programs of conduct, such as medical training curricula, and what Foucault calls the "codifying effects" of knowledge about various therapies, populations, and validity measurements: "The production of true discourses served to found, justify, and provide reasons and principles for these ways of doing things" (252).

The statements found in an archive are understood as answers to emerging questions and as solutions to emerging problems in a discursive field. Genealogical research aims to identify these "problematizations": "To analyze problematizations is to investigate why certain things (behaviour, phenomena, processes) become articulated *as* problems, how they are linked up with or divided off from other phenomena, and the various ways (conditions and procedures) in which this actually happens" (Osborne and Rose 1997, 97, emphasis in original; cf. Foucault 1988, 17). For instance, over the last half of the twentieth century, Western medicine became specifically concerned with questions about the nature of clinical practice. Archival statements about clinical practice represent "styles of articulation," which are "a way of giving voice to a certain set of problems and aspirations." EBM is a result not only of efforts to scientifically systematize and classify clinical judgments but also of questions about the application of scientific research to clinical practice. Each of these developments can be traced through the changing problematizations of medical practice, which are the "conditions for the emergence of new theories" (Osborne and Rose 1997, 88). In other words, EBM is a product of the social and historical circumstances that enabled the articulation of a set of problems relating to clinical judgment in the research literature, and these articulations served to found, justify, and provide reasons for the reform of medical practice.

The statements in archival documents were created in institutional spaces. In his historical work, Foucault explains both the practices and events that relocated the medical gaze onto the human body: the study of medical discourse was carried out "*in a field of non-discursive practices*" (Foucault 1972, 68, emphasis in original). Nondiscursive practices are "characterized by the demarcation of a field of objects, by the definition of a legitimate perspective for a subject of knowledge, by the setting of norms for elaborating concepts and theories. Hence, each of them presupposes a play of prescriptions that govern exclusions and selections" (Foucault 1994, 11). I see the field of EBM as bringing together both ways of knowing and prescriptive rules for doctors to follow, such as diagnosing illnesses (e.g., diagnostic criteria, reading test results) and recommending therapies (e.g., writing prescriptions). Osborne (1992, 79) refers to Foucault's notion of the medical gaze as follows: "This mode of problematization concerns, above all, the way that forms of knowledge, vision and enunciation are articulated together into a particular perceptual model; a kind of 'sensory economy' that articulates what the doctor can see, feel, say, teach, or know, and which brings about more or less of an alignment of these functions." My objective is to demonstrate how these relations of discourse aligned with certain forms of conduct (i.e., what people see, say, and do, and the rules associated with these practices).

I collected archival statements that problematized medical practices associated with clinical judgment. These statements articulated, in the words of historical sociologist Mitchell Dean (1994, 195), the "different ways in which being is necessarily given to thought and the practices that give form to thought." EBM determines what kinds of knowledge and statements are considered true within the clinic, and what kinds of knowledge and statements are considered false. When analyzing a document, my task is not to merely interpret its meaning; rather, I seek to examine how discourse "organises the document, divides it up, distributes it, orders, arranges it in levels, establishes series, distinguishes between what is relevant and what is not, discovers elements, defines unities, describes relations" (Foucault 1972, 6–7). I do not use documents to reconstruct the past (cf. Dean 1994, 15), but, instead, to locate "problematizations through which being offers itself to be, necessarily, thought – and the *practices* on the basis of which these problematizations are formed" (Foucault 1985, 11, emphasis in original). In this way, I examine how certain kinds of practices became problematic within the field of medicine.

After my archival visits, I coded documents for what they had to say about clinical judgment. To paraphrase Rose and Miller (1992, 177), the significance of medical discourse is not treated as a top-down ideology; rather, it helps to elucidate not only the systems of thought that articulated the problems of clinical medicine but also the systems of action through which the institution of medicine has sought to remedy those problems. I examine documents for both their scientific statements about clinical judgment as a problematic object and for the solutions offered to correct the identified issues. I take systems of knowledge to be more than just ideas that individuals wrote down; rather, I view them as an "assemblage of persons, theories, projects, experiments and techniques" (Rose and Miller 1992, 177). My archive is composed of statements made by a variety of actors within the social field of medicine, from individual clinicians who were encountering problems in their practice, to ministers of health and education, to university presidents and teachers, among others. The problems of medicine are posed on many terrains, from theories of ecology to logic and decision theory to laboratory medical sciences. The projects that aimed to correct for these problems associated with clinical judgment include new school curricula and new scientific measurements. I observe that the deployment of this knowledge serves to justify the disciplinary techniques that regulate the responsibility of clinicians to keep pace with the most up-to-date evidence.

My research does not attempt to update the visualities of Foucault's argument on the discursive link between seeing and saying.[4] Rather, my genealogical approach takes a direction that differs from that taken in Foucault's work on the medical field. In the words of Osborne (1992, 64), *The Birth of the Clinic* was not about a professional monopoly of knowledge: "The 'profession' monopolizes knowledge in a closed domain – whilst a further gesture of exclusion takes place, within the profession, through the malign development of 'specialization.'" In fact, Foucault spends hardly any time on the role of force relations in organizing medical activity. His focus was far more archeological than genealogical, but the latter implies archaeology in that it requires researchers to investigate the "conditions of existence" that relate discourse to "the practical field in which it is applied" (Foucault 1991, 60–61). My research begins by considering the relations of discourse, and then I shift my analysis to the conditions that shaped the reorganization of medical activity. In the words of Jon Frauley (2007, 626), I examine EBM discourse "as a structure that is emergent from conditions and which can produce effects in the practical field in which it is employed." Foucault's early work on medicine contains no mention of the form of power that, in *Discipline and Punish,* he came to refer to as "normalization" (cf. Osborne 1992, 72), which can be understood as the use of scientifically established standards to regulate human activity in institutionally installed programs of conduct. I am updating Foucault's work on medicine by making connections between the discursive practices of knowing and the normalizing regulatory mechanisms of the profession of medicine. I explain not just where EBM came from but also what relations of power mobilize medical knowledge, how it came to organize certain forms of activity, and why it continues despite being an impossible project.

From Strategy to Dispositif
In order to support my claim that EBM has stabilized within a dispositif, I now explain how I used Foucault's criteria. "Dispositif" is a French word often translated as "apparatus,"[5] and it is defined as

a thoroughly heterogenous ensemble consisting of discourses, institutions, architectural forms, regulatory decisions, laws, administrative measures, scientific statements, philanthropic proposition – in short, the said as much as the unsaid. Such are the elements of the apparatus. The apparatus itself is the system of relations that can be established between these elements." (Foucault 1980b, 194)

The apparatus of medicine is made up of an assemblage of various parts, including particular institutions (such as the McMaster University medical school and the colleges of physicians and surgeons); architectural forms (such as the health sciences complex, built to train new medical school graduates at McMaster); regulatory decisions (such as curriculum development and disciplinary committees in medical colleges); and scientific statements (such as clinical epidemiology). I investigate these various elements, all of which coalesce around the discourse of EBM, and the relations of normalization and discipline that structure them.

In order for EBM to go on, despite concerns about its present crisis, this apparatus must be strategic by nature: "In order for a certain relation of forces not only to maintain itself, but to accentuate, stabilise and broaden itself, a certain kind of manoeuvre is necessary" (Foucault 1980b, 206). Apparatuses emerge historically in response to an "urgent need": this is the element of problematization. Clinical epidemiology, and later EBM, emerge in medical discourse at the precise moment that the discursive object of clinical judgment is under scrutiny from within and beyond medicine. As a solution installed in a particular institution, the apparatus, according to Foucault, "has a dominant strategic function" (195). The historical emergence of EBM was contingent on the need to rework medical training and practice (what Foucault calls functional overdetermination) after various challenges to medical practice in the mid-twentieth century. The strategic elaboration of EBM aimed to allow physicians to critically appraise evidence and apply it at the bedside; however, it also produced unintended effects, such as deresponsibilization.

EBM has become the dominant model of Western medicine because its knowledge and techniques of regulation serve as tactics to enable the persistence of overarching liberal strategies of

governance. Strategies of domination are defined via the following assumptions:

> Domination is organised into a more-or-less coherent and uni-
> tary strategic form; that dispersed, heteromorphous, localized
> procedures of power are adapted, re-enforced and transformed
> by these global strategies, all this being accompanied by num-
> erous phenomena of inertia, displacement and resistance; hence
> one should not assume a massive and primal condition of dom-
> ination, a binary structure with "dominators" on one side and
> "dominated" on the other, but rather a multiform production of
> relations of domination which are partially susceptible of inte-
> gration into overall strategies. (Foucault 1980b, 142)

To illustrate the above, Canadian politicians are able to benefit
from the responsibilizing and individualizing disciplinary techniques of the medical colleges. It is not that politicians have carefully worked out some project to save money by off-loading the
improvement of health care onto physicians and medical colleges.
Rather, the current assemblage of EBM and medical colleges
serves to maintain the dominant way of governing – one that uses
as little regulation as possible at the least possible cost. In politics,
in order to maintain power it is advantageous to spend as little as
possible on health care and to provide tax cuts. Foucault uses a
similar form of analysis in *Discipline and Punish* when he shows
that not only are criminals not reformed by prisons but, on their
release, their marginalization within society as ex-convicts renders
them "useful" to the bourgeoisie and their tolerated illegalities
(see my discussion on pp. 174–75).

Foucault's model is not meant to provide a normative critique,
but it does explain how the effects of any institution can be used
to further perpetuate the dominant relations of ruling. Medical
colleges deploy disciplinary techniques to dominate and correct
poor decisions made by physicians. Thus, the concept of tactics
is defined as "the art of constructing, with located bodies, coded
activities and trained aptitudes, mechanisms in which the product

of the various forces is increased by their calculated combination" (Foucault 1979, 166). Strategies, then, aim to align the effects of tactics, such as disciplinary techniques, with the objective of supporting the overall strategy of domination. The strategies of liberal governance maintain domination by organizing the deresponsibilizing effect produced by medical colleges that use evidence-based CPGs to discipline physicians.

Chapter Overview

I conceptualize the apparatus of medicine as "inscribed in a play of power," to paraphrase Foucault (1980a, 196), "but it is also always linked to certain coordinates of knowledge which issue from it but, to an equal degree, condition it." Given that an apparatus consists of "strategies of relations of forces supporting, and supported by, types of knowledge" (ibid.), I first seek to analyze those strategies that structure the field of EBM. In "La pussière et les nuage" Foucault (1980a) spells out his method for analyzing strategies through genealogical analysis. The researcher examines the following elements: the formation of discursive relations; the genesis of knowledge and tactics that individuals apply in determining how to conduct themselves as well as how to judge and instruct the conduct of others; and why these tactics were chosen rather than others. The researcher does this in order to determine what effects have occurred (including disorders, damage, and/ or unforeseen and uncontrolled consequences) due to the application of these strategies and how their failure has led to their reconsideration. I now provide the layout of my argument, which moves from a genealogy of clinical epidemiology, to EBM, to the programs of conduct that come to regulate medical activity, to the consequences that follow.

Mykhalovskiy and Weir (2004) argue that social science research has not paid enough attention to the question of EBM – specifically, its impact on the medical profession and the transformation of biomedical reasoning and practices. They suggest that social scientists examine the "discursive preconditions" of

EBM and ask what questions led to the emergence of clinical epidemiology: "How the apparent oxymoron, clinical epidemiology, became historically possible and to what it was a solution is a topic in need of a genealogy" (Mykhalovskiy and Weir 2004, 1065). My research begins by considering the concerns to which clinical epidemiology (and later EBM) was a solution, and how this form of knowledge is used to regulate human activity in the clinic. Chapter 1 works through the discursive relations of EBM. I explore the medical literature in order to spell out how certain questions about the nature of clinical judgments emerged post-Second World War. I draw on an archival analysis of medical journals that were published in Western medicine to show that clinical judgments were rendered visible as the site of a problem that had to be ameliorated. I show the role of clinical epidemiology, an emerging science in the latter half of the twentieth century, in formulating the problems of medical practice as something that could be remedied through educational reform. Chapter 1 spells out the conditions of possibility for seeing clinical judgments as problematic aspects of human activity in the clinic. It sets up the argument in the following chapter, which explains the genesis of this knowledge and how the tactics of conduct changed medical practice. I also discuss alternate and unsuccessful solutions to the identified problems as well as the discursive mechanisms that continue to reproduce those same problems in the present discourse. On finishing this chapter, readers should understand how clinical epidemiology, and later EBM, emerged from questions surrounding the nature of clinical judgment and the desire to control it.

Chapter 2 explores the material relations that organize human activity, and it does so by spelling out the historical, political, and economic conditions that allowed particular changes to medical training programs to occur in lieu of other possibilities. I show how the problematization of clinical judgment in the clinical epidemiology literature provided a justification for creating a new method of training medical students at McMaster University. I draw on archival materials from the government, McMaster University, and the National Archives to show how the McMaster health centre facilities reorganized medical practice. I also touch on Canada's contribution to the present methods of medical training and practice. On finishing this chapter, readers should understand the material relations that both organized the new model of medical training and contributed to its success in Canada and abroad.

Chapter 3 builds on the work of Chapter 2 and extends the case study of the McMaster medical school by providing an analysis of the development of tactics for conducting oneself and judging the conduct of others. Problem-based learning is a method of instruction that was pioneered at McMaster. Its underlying principles focus on training students how to integrate knowledge into practice through applying a specific method of problem solving. This method is understood as a technique that individualizes students as responsible for their own learning, and it is justified by a pedagogy that aims to ameliorate the identified problems of clinical practice. I draw on archival materials from the government, McMaster University, and the Royal College of Physicians and Surgeons of Canada to show how the McMaster curriculum made it possible to reconceptualize the responsibility of physicians to keep up with knowledge production and, in so doing, opened up new opportunities for medical regulation. On finishing this chapter, readers should understand how problem-based learning responsibilized the newly conceived student of medical education.

Chapter 4 links changes in medical education with emerging methods for regulating physicians once they have completed their training. Regulation is, according to Rose and Miller (1992, 181) a "problematizing activity" – it seeks to identify the problems of medicine, which have been predominantly associated with clinical judgment. The regulatory programs that articulate what is desirable – the use of evidence in practice – aim to intervene in a way that is viable: "Programmes ... make the objects of government thinkable in such a way that their ills appear susceptible to diagnosis, prescription and cure by calculating and normalizing intervention" (183). EBM emphasizes the use of the best evidence in clinical practice. But, as spelled out in the medical literature, evidence and science are always changing – plus, there is so much evidence that it is difficult to know which would best inform clinical decision making. EBM allowed CPGs to become an important part of medical practice. I show how national collaborations between the government and the Canadian Medical Association (CMA) have changed how the medical profession regulates its practitioners. Medical licensing colleges across Canada endorse CPGs and encourage their use in medical practice. By engaging with data from a study of medical disciplinary actions across Canada, I show the effects of the apparatus of EBM, specifically arguing that guidelines are used to regulate physicians. I explain how CPGs are used in medical regulation to normalize professional judgments in the clinic, and this externalizes the judgments of individual practitioners – an effect that I term "deresponsibilization." This concept is a new contribution to the sociology of medicine. On finishing this chapter, readers should understand not only how EBM allowed CPGs to become the norm in the medical profession but also how CPGs act on the subjectivity of practitioners.

Chapter 5, "The Impossible Clinic," seeks to explain how the strategic effects of EBM – specifically, deresponsibilization – have been utilized to perpetuate relations of domination. To do this I shift from examining the disciplinary techniques and normalizing relations of the medical colleges to examining the relations of force that allow EBM to keep going despite its antithetical effects on clinical subjectivity and its failure to meet its objectives. Individualizing the problems of health care and reducing them to the judgment of clinicians defines the problem of medicine within the clinic, which, in turn, determines the juridical elements of the policy programs installed in medical education and regulation. Despite the failed effects, this diverts attention away from the potential failure of health infrastructure and focuses it on individual decisions, which require amelioration. These effects are consistent with advanced liberal principles of rule. I conclude by explaining how the concept of responsibilization and Rose's notion of "ethopolitics" in the sociology of health and medicine are based on the assumption that individuals "choose to work on themselves" and that they make decisions through addressing a series of choices about how they ought to make judgments about their health. I make an original contribution to governmentality studies and the sociology of medicine in that I show how professional governance strategies in medicine may not require doctors to "think": rather, they should follow rules, and this represents a failure of professional governance strategies within liberal governmentality. Professional regulation has an effect on responsibility within medicine, and this deserves further attention and research.

The conclusion links Foucauldian genealogy with the sociology of medicine. I close by considering the transformative possibilities of genealogy through a discussion of Foucault's notion of the specific intellectual and how to practise public sociology in the sociology of medicine.

1

Conversations in Medicine:
Problematizing Clinical Practice

IN THIS CHAPTER I discuss six problems in the medical literature that led to the first statements of evidence-based medicine. I locate the strategic relations of discourse and explain the discursive conditions that problematized clinical judgment. It was from the articulation of a number of "problems" in clinical practice that the object of clinical judgment became the juridical target of programmatic intervention. The narrative begins with questions surrounding the laboratory and medical research as well as the clinic and the health of patients. Although other important literature examines the role of the "therapeutic revolution," such as the development of new drugs and the role of the state in the regulation of health care,[1] my goal is to show how a justification for the scientific study of clinical judgments emerged from concerns about the applicability of laboratory research to doctors' individual practices. The questions that problematize clinical practice led to new methods for reforming and systematizing medical training.

Following Foucault, my sociological analytic visualizes medicine as a discursive terrain, a formation of various relations that structure and make possible what people do and say in a given practice. During his archaeological period, Foucault (1972, 67) defined the relations of discourse as a discursive formation:

This whole group of relations forms a principle of determination that permits or excludes, within a given discourse, a certain number of statements: these are conceptual systematizations, enunciative series, groups and organizations of objects that might have been possible (and of which nothing can justify the absence at the level of their own rules of formation), but which are excluded by a discursive constellation at a higher level and in a broader space.

In assuming this definition, I conceptualize EBM as a discursive formation that conceptualizes and stipulates which judgments are evidence-based in the clinic and which are not. The relations of discourse form what can and cannot be considered scientific about the field of medical practice. In the words of Jon Frauley (2007, 626), a "'discursive formation' is just such a field in which action, indirect mechanisms and techniques, socio-political objects, regulatory objects and authorities emerge." The condition of possibility for making a statement about the nature of a particular disease, for example, depends on the epistemological rules for defining it on the body. *The Birth of the Clinic* documents the emergence of a specific set of rules for seeing disease on the body: "The space of configuration of the disease and the space of localization of the illness in the body have been superimposed, in medical experience, for only a relatively short period of time" (Foucault 1973a, 3). Foucault analyzed a number of events that changed the discursive field of medicine in the nineteenth century and, subsequently, its object. In this chapter, I expand on Foucault's earlier conception of medicine by first describing the relations of discourse and then explaining how they functioned to problematize clinical judgment in the field of medicine.

I operationalize the relations of discourse by analyzing "the strategic apparatus which permits of separating out from among all the statements which are possible those that will be acceptable within, I won't say a scientific theory, but a field of scientificity, and which it is possible to say are true or false." I argue that the field of clinical epidemiology became the dominant discursive formation; it became the solution to the identified problems of clinical judgment, and it permitted the field of clinical medicine to be "scientific." The relations of discourse "makes possible the separation, not of the true from the false, but of what may from what may not be characterized as scientific" (Foucault 1980b, 197). I locate and analyze the relations of discourse that came to problematize and later resolve the identified problems associated with clinical judgment in order to show how these relations have become predominant in medicine and how, later, they served to justify the organization of medical training.

The Laboratory and the Clinic

Historical research has shown that clinical epidemiology emerged as an answer to growing concerns and questions about the role of laboratory medicine (i.e., research) and its applicability to (or incompatibility with) bedside practices. Biomedicine emerged as the dominant science of medicine and medical education after the Second World War. Biomedicine is an approach to medicine that allows "knowledge creators" (e.g., teachers, researchers, textbook authors, and so on) to use the scientific paradigm in both knowledge-production and medical training systems (Kleinman 1997). According to historian Jeanne Daly (2005, 42), during the 1950s the laboratory was the centre of medical knowledge: "The laboratory became the focus for research, and the laboratory moved into the hospital next to patients. Increasingly the laboratory became the principal source of information for purposes of diagnosis and the main source of understanding the nature of disease." During a time of rapid change, increasing innovations, and technological developments, there were questions about the relationship between the biomedical sciences and health care practices.[2] These concerns led to new approaches to medical practice. For example, White, Williams, and Greenberg (1961, 885) refer to the "ecology of medical care" as an approach that aimed to reduce the disjuncture between technological improvements and research advances in the laboratory with a "measurable improvement in the health of a society's member" (891). In other words, there were concerns over whether the improvements in science could be measured in terms of improving the health of individual patients. If improvements could not be measured, the authors wondered, on what basis would it be possible to reform the whole institution of medicine?

Alongside these questions about the relationship between the effectiveness of medicine and population health there appeared the field of clinical epidemiology. Clinical epidemiology aimed to generate knowledge about clinical practice, specifically by examining the clinician's judgment. During the 1960s, questions arose about the authority of medical knowledge: How much authority does the doctor's individual judgment have? Alvan Feinstein describes the emergence of this problem in relation to his own individual experience as a doctor participating in a broad epidemiological study of population health and rheumatic fever.[3] As part of a medical study, Feinstein listened to the heartbeat of participating patients to determine whether there was a murmur, which might indicate a condition. While listening to a patient's heart, he heard a faint murmur that had not been recorded in the patient's medical history. He realized that, had he not heard it, it would have affected the patient's future health, and he further wondered if he had made similar mistakes in the past with other patients. Feinstein associated this problem with the nature of clinical judgment. He set out to eliminate the variations that resulted from the physician's interpretation of symptoms on the patient's body. In *Clinical Judgment,* Feinstein describes how to use scientific taxonomy to minimize discrepancies in diagnosis and variation in health care. He intended to improve the practice of clinical judgments and medical practice: "What choices would doctors really be confident about? Honest, dedicated clinicians today disagree on the treatment for almost every disease from the common cold to the metastatic cancer. Our experiments in treatment were acceptable by the standards of the community, but were not reproducible by the standards of science" (Feinstein 1967, 14).

Feinstein proposed a method for applying scientific criteria to judgments made in the clinic. He argued that patients needed to be classified in relation to a larger population because, due to the ranges of variance in the categories of the classification, it was difficult to diagnose an illness in an individual patient. Classification, he reasoned, would provide accurate comparisons between populations and a scientific basis for applying therapeutic interventions to similar populations (Feinstein 1967, 227). Once patients could be classified in relation to their disease behaviour, they could be plotted on a distribution of population variance in order to render some plausible scientific knowledge about care interventions. The way to implement this change, Feinstein claimed, was for physicians to study their own practice, to "observe it accurately, classify it, and use it to determine prognosis and guide treatment" (quoted in Daly 2005, 31).

Feinstein anticipated what would become the prevalent anxiety of the medical field in the following decade: the scientific basis of care and medical authority. His writing reflects a dominant problematization of the clinician's judgment, primarily through a formulation of the objectivity of the physician's interpretation of the clinical evidence. Feinstein (1967, 28) suggests that the pace of technological and therapeutic advances in medicine had overtaken the current methods of clinical judgments: "The intellectual technology of clinical judgment – the methods of acquiring evidence and organizing clinical thought – has not received the same attention that contemporary clinical scientists have given to chemical, mechanical, electronic, and other new inanimate methods for observing and assessing tangible materials." These scientific advancements in medicine led to concerns over their benefit for the health of the population overall and, more particularly, over the physician's authority. The changing world of medicine led to practical problems for medical practitioners who were beginning to wonder about the relationship between research and practice, biomedical science and bedside care: "Therapeutic decisions ... [are] scientifically unapproachable because they depend on clinical and personal data obtained and analyzed by one human being observing other human beings" (29). The basis for the clinician's assessment of medical "data," or evidence, was under scrutiny, and the field of medicine required a scientific basis for everyday practice.

The establishment of a problematization often occurs in institutional contexts: "[Problematization] show[s] that at each moment a precise set of problems were the target of thought and action, within certain specific practices, and that a given problematization was first of all an answer given by definite individuals in specific texts, although it may later come to be so general as to become anonymous" (Osborne and Rose 1997, 94; cf. Foucault 1988, 17). For Feinstein, those problems concerned the ability of the clinician to systematically interpret clinical evidence and combine it with other observable factors. He proposed to remedy the problems related to the subjective aspects of care with the values and principles of the scientific method, its objectivity and its commitments to reproducibility. Doing so, he reasoned, could eliminate the uncertainties that resulted from variation. These interventions focused on the capacity of the clinician's judgment. His concerns with the link between scientific principles of clinical practice and the patient would later be taken up and dealt with through the establishment of the discipline of clinical epidemiology.

At the time that Feinstein's *Clinical Judgment* was published in 1967, David Sackett, who would later become known as part of the EBM Working Group, was leading the first department of clinical epidemiology at McMaster University. Sackett was influenced by Feinstein's *Clinical Judgment,* and he later published an article about the importance of the emerging field of clinical epidemiology. He defined the clinical epidemiologist as "an individual with extensive training and experience in clinical medicine who, after receiving appropriate training in epidemiology and biostatistics, *continues to provide direct patient care* in his subsequent career" (Sackett 1969, 125, emphasis added). He justified the need for such a field by citing the overspecialization of statisticians in biometric modelling who lacked proficiency in the problems encountered by practising clinicians (ibid.). He recommended the reform of medical education and training in order to provide clinicians with the skills to ask epidemiological questions relevant to immediate clinical practice (127). Later, I examine Sackett's recommendations with regard to medical education, reform, and the significance and relevance of epidemiological knowledge in clinical practice.

The authority of the clinician's judgment continued to be problematized in medicine through the following decade. Questions arose from both outside and inside the medical field. A discussion of medical authority further demonstrates the problematization of clinical judgment, something that could later provide the basis for the juridical solution to these problems – the reform of medical training.

Questioning Medical Authority: Clinical Authority, Subjective Morality, Practice Variation

In the 1970s, the medical profession was challenged to account for the basis of clinical judgments, the role of the doctor's subjective morality, and practice variation. Medical professionals began to ask about the validity of "using traditional clinical authority as the basis for clinical decision making" (Daly 2005, 1). The introduction of laboratory and medical sciences to clinical practice was thought to be a solution to the "traditional," or conventional, authority of the doctor. The medical paternalism of "doctor knows best" could not stand up to questions about hard facts: How does the doctor know what to diagnose or prescribe? Where did that knowledge come from? Intuition? Somewhere else? The introduction of scientific methods to primary care depended on this link between medical research and the clinic.

In the annual oration of the Massachusetts Medical Society,[4] Donnell W. Boardman (1974, 502) stated: "In a time of medical priesthoods the doctor-patient relation was primarily the responsibility of the physician ... In the era of the scientific method the physician has learned to look critically at the case and at its component parts, a valuable and useful process that has nonetheless separated the medical scientist from the sick person." The link between science and clinical judgment was again presented as a solution to growing changes within medical practice. Boardman noted that changes in technology played a role in the questions surrounding the scientific basis of clinical care: technology was increasingly being used, but, he argued, physicians were in need of knowing when a situation would call for the use of new technology, why new developments were needed, and how this might affect the health of the patient.

There was also a concern among medical students about the relationship between medicine and other institutions. As McNamara (1972) explains, the students in medical schools during the 1960s were the students of social change, involved in protest movements concerning human rights. McNamara saw the next generation of medical students as one that sought to reconnect the clinic with the community, not the laboratory. He documented the concerns of newly minted physicians who were feeling isolated in their practice, and he called on them to be more involved in community and researcher (laboratory) partnerships in order to produce better methods for their clinical practice. Students, he argued, saw medicine as a rapidly changing field, with new technologies emerging exponentially after the war, and they wanted to be a part of the revolution. The significance of medical authority and the outcomes of clinical care can be observed in these student concerns. Medical practice relies on interacting with members of one's community and making decisions about patients that may result in either life or death. However, the interest in having some justifiable knowledge about what medicine could offer would later be resolved via the assumptions and evidence of science. The interest in reconnecting with the community was marginalized by the concerns of clinical epidemiology and its emphasis on forming connections with science and technology. In order to bring together assumptions and evidence within the clinic, the clinician's judgment would become the target of training and reform.

Medical authority was also called into question by studies from other human sciences. Social science research turned its interests to the professions, including medicine. The social perception of medicine was changing. For example, in 1967, David Sudnow published a study about death in the emergency room.

He reported that the designation of clinical death depended on the attending physician's moral perception of the patient. Those who were deemed "clinically dead" by doctors were considered to be "potentially revivable" (Sudnow 1967, 37). Younger people were more likely to be revived than old, and those who died at their own hands or by "stupidity" were less likely to receive special attention for resuscitation. Sudnow's documentation of these variances in care demonstrated that medical practice, despite common perceptions, was not objective: clinicians attached *subjective* meaning to a patient's life, and they oriented the execution of their actions (e.g., decision to resuscitate) in light of broader cultural significance rather than science. How could members of the public know whether the care they received was coming from an objective physician or from a physician who was applying her/his own morality?

A study conducted by Wennberg and Gittelsohn (1973) documents regional variations in the delivery of medical care. Their study, published in *Science,* shows that doctors treated patients with the same diagnosis in different ways and that this could be observed by region. Similar to Sudnow's study, Wennberg and Gittelsohn's work disturbs the assumption that what doctors learned in medical school was a body of knowledge and a set of procedures that ensured that all patients with the same ailments would receive the same treatment. Further, who could say that the doctors in one region were providing better care than the doctors in another region? These two exemplary studies are signposts indicating the emerging problematization of individual physicians and their judgments. Questions about the basis of medical practice were raised both in medicine and in other disciplines. Medicine would answer these questions by producing new theories and measurements to eliminate practice variation. It would appeal to the authority of science to resolve these issues, and the judgments of clinicians would come to be the site for intervention: morality and variance would come to be understood as individualized problems that could be corrected through better training.

Establishing New Measurements

The randomized controlled trial (RCT) has become what EBM considers the "gold standard" for valid knowledge about effective treatments and therapies (Sackett et al. 2000). During the 1970s, Archibald Cochrane's postwar research modified the RCT by introducing controlled groups to patient trials in order to increase the reliability and validity of trial results (Daly 2005, 131–32). The RCT is a method of testing a medical intervention according to which a patient population is randomized into two groups: one that receives the treatment and one that does not (the "control group"). The progress of the disease is measured by comparing the results of those not receiving the treatment with the results of those receiving the treatment. The success of the therapy or intervention is subject to statistical analysis to determine the effect of the treatment. The results of RCTs often generate recommendations about the efficacy of medical therapies.[5]

The RCT is considered to be the offspring of a 1940s clinical trial conducted by Austin Bradford Hill that tested the effects of streptomycin, a treatment for tuberculosis. In 1946, one clinic in the United Kingdom only had enough of the therapy to treat fifty patients, which was far fewer than the number infected. So, at the time, Hill, the attending physician, thought it would be unethical to do anything but a *randomized* clinical trial among the patients in his population (Chalmers 2001). The results of Hill's research were published in 1948 (Hill 1948). His method was modified by Archibald Cochrane's postwar research through the introduction of controlled groups to patient trials (Daly 2005, 131–32).

Iain Chalmers, a student of Cochrane, spent much of his career arguing for new methodologies in health, specifically in his sub-specialty field of perinatal research. His approach would come to influence the proliferation of new technologies. His early research focused on the inadequacy of measurement indices for understanding risk in his field (e.g., Chalmers 1979). One of the major criticisms Chalmers launched against clinical practice concerned its unsystematic use of experimentation: "The idea that doctors conduct poorly controlled, uninterpretable experiments daily comes as a jolt to most patients. In individual doctor-patient encounters, frank discussion of uncertainty has been rare" (Chalmers and Silverman 1987, 388–89). One of his major contributions to medicine was his focus on defending and promoting the use of evidence from RCTs to eliminate unsystematic experimentation in clinical medicine.

Following Cochrane, Chalmers wanted to eliminate bias in medical studies in order to improve the evidence derived from medical sciences and make it more applicable to the clinic. For example, Cochrane saw perinatal medicine as the least scientific field of clinical practice: most of its studies had insufficient evidence for the recommendations that they made to clinicians. The randomized double-blind trial, Chalmers argued, would eliminate selection and measurement bias (Chalmers 1984, 722). As a response to these concerns, Chalmers, along with Canadian physician and researcher Murray Enkin, embarked on the task of creating the Oxford Database of Perinatal Trials, the first database to contain a collection of RCT studies relating to the field of obstetrics. The goals of the initiative were to provide a register for RCTs in the perinatal field in order "to encourage a scientifically based approach to the care of mothers and babies" (Chalmers et al. 1986, 307). Doing so, they hoped, would improve the quality of care: it was "a vast task of collating and synthesizing studies (mainly randomized controlled trials) into systematic reviews" (Daly 2005, 7). They recommended that other specialties form their own databases for similar purposes.

In addition to the RCT, another new method that aimed to eliminate clinical problems was the systematic review. Systematic reviews are secondary research, and they synthesize the findings from all available RCTs on therapeutic intervention. Chalmers was instrumental in establishing this method within the relations of discourse. Along with colleagues, he argued that new research in medicine failed "to apply scientific principles in their discussions of how the newly generated evidence accords with previously available information" (Chalmers, Enkin, and Keirse 1993, 411). The authors laid out a series of procedures for producing systematic reviews that could compare studies with different populations, interventions, study designs, and so on, in an attempt to reduce error and bias while also synthesizing new knowledge with existing clinical practices. In 1992, the initiative would lead to the creation of the Cochrane Collaboration, named for Archibald Cochrane.[6] The Cochrane Collaboration was a database of RCTs and systematic reviews to which creators and users could gain access and then assess evidence. Paraphrasing Cochrane's own *Effectiveness and Efficiency*, the authors justified the creation of the Cochrane database with the following words: "Extensive worldwide collaboration is required to accomplish the task of synthesizing existing information about the effects of health care efficiently. And efficiency is essential. People using the health services have already waited too long for the available evidence to be assembled and kept up to date" (425–26).

By 1994, there were hundreds of researchers contributing to the Cochrane Collaboration from myriad institutions worldwide (Chalmers and Haynes 1994, 863). The goal was to expand the focus of the project to include as many areas of medical practice as possible, using electronic distribution as a fast way to create and update systematic reviews as research continued to emerge. By 1995, Chalmers had linked his initiative with the EBM discourse, calling the collaboration an effort in the "development of evidence-based health care" (67). It was argued that the Cochrane database provided access to systematic reviews and that these were better than single studies because, given that the database synthesized the results of one study with all existing evidence, they were able to assess the quality of evidence in relation to clinical practice. The authority of the physician's judgment could be validated by recourse to the best available research on the effectiveness of tested medical interventions. This was one initiative that aimed to resolve the problems associated with individual interpretations of evidence by giving physicians information to use in their practice.

In addition to the establishment of the RCT and the systematic review as the best forms of evidence in the order of discourse, the introduction of Bayesian logic in the 1970s was another new development regarding questions about the measures of scientific validity in the clinic. Bayesian logic was brought into philosophy as a way to calculate whether a hypothesis is true given the available evidence. It evaluates the probability of later events given events that have already occurred and that have been observed. In other words, given certain evidence, the philosopher can determine if their hypothesis is supported based on prior probabilities. In the clinical setting, Bayes's theorem was considered helpful for marrying the objective knowledge from the laboratory to the clinical expertise (subjective experience) of the physician. Diagnoses and prognoses, for example, could be made based on *both* the physician's subjective criteria and the "diagnostic probability" *and* the statistical likelihood that a therapy would work on a particular patient. Henrik R. Wulff's (1976, 3) *Rational Diagnosis and Treatment* explains the benefits of Bayesian logic for drawing "practical conclusions from the research of others":

It is necessary but not sufficient that the clinician has a thorough nosological knowledge. He will not become a good diagnostician, until he has learnt to estimate correctly the incidence of different diseases and the incidence of different disease manifestations among his patients. Bayes' theorem is the mathematical illustration of the concept of diagnostic experience. (84)

Bayes's theorem provided a way to determine the probability of some clinical judgments (e.g., diagnoses) over others given biological evidence (objective) and clinical experience (subjective). The doctor's "hypothesis" about diagnosis or treatment could be validated in relation to prior evidence, which could come from population observations (such as those from clinical trials). The problems associated with clinical evidence could be reduced via these logical procedures. Subsequently, decisions about the likely outcomes of various treatment programs depended on an accurate diagnosis. This logic would later inform EBM. The importance of attaining the correct diagnosis is crucial to effective evidence-based practice. Statistical measurements of probability were articulated as solutions to identified problems with clinical judgments insofar as subjective knowledge could be justified by the principles of science. These new methods of reasoning emerged within the new discourse of clinical epidemiology, and they formed the scientific basis for reforms in medical education that would train physicians to use scientific reasoning to make better clinical judgments.

Reforming Medical Education

There were other concerns in the medical literature about medical education: new technologies demanded new educational formats (e.g., Waugh 1984, 145). Student representatives who served on medical association councils also wanted more rigid guidelines for certification (e.g., Davis 1981, 1194). Other physicians discussed reforming the curriculum in order to instill clinicians with certain characteristics rather than with knowledge per se (e.g., Light 1979, 320).

Starting in the 1980s, some medical school training programs began to make clinical epidemiology a mandatory course for medical students. Students resisted epidemiology courses because they were statistically and mathematically complex. Yet historians of medicine's recent past have found evidence that students also wanted to know how to make clinical decisions with certainty (e.g., see Daly 2005, 23). In their book, Bursztajn and colleagues (1981) detail a "clash" of old and new "paradigms" of medical practice. The old paradigm was the laboratory scientist who looked for hard evidence for objective decisions. The new paradigm was the next generation of physicians – people who were interested in probabilities and recognized that all decisions are made in the face of uncertainty (see also Pease 1981, 1731).

One of the first textbooks for medical school courses in clinical epidemiology was written by Fletcher, Fletcher, and Wagner, who were researchers at the University of North Carolina. They define clinical epidemiology as the application of "epidemiologic principles and methods to problems encountered in clinical medicine." They go on to say, "it is a science concerned with counting clinical events occurring in intact human beings, and it uses epidemiologic methods to carry out and analyze the count" (Fletcher, Fletcher, and Wagner 1982, 2). Fletcher and colleagues also discuss the problems of medical authority and the scientific solution:

> Sometimes we [students] were comfortable taking the word of a trusted authority. But the limitations of this approach were apparent. For one thing, experts often disagree and so could not all be right. Not only did they disagree about the wisdom of a given diagnostic or therapeutic approach, but also about the validity of the evidence upon which their recommendations were based. Also, most faculty were involved in laboratory research and found it difficult to apply the kind of scientific approaches used in the laboratory to the solution of clinical problems. Evidence that could not be reduced to "hard science" was sometimes viewed by them with uncertainty and suspicion. (vii)

In the preface to their book, they problematize clinical judgment as a rationale for the reform of medical education, including the questioning of medical authority and the relevance of laboratory research to clinical practice. In addition to discussing a variety of important issues in clinical epidemiology, their basic argument is that medical students should critically analyze and appraise the evidence they encounter in medical journals in order to make decisions about which data and evidence are valid and relevant in clinical practice (217). The solution to the problems within the literature required individuals to learn better decision making methods, which, in turn, rendered clinical judgments more scientific. Later, I discuss critical appraisal as central to the link between clinical epidemiology and the establishment of EBM.

Justifying the New Science of Clinical Care

In light of the changing landscape of medical practice and education, discussions between medical researchers and physicians concerning the scientific nature of clinical practice continued into the

1980s. There was an increasing interest in studying clinical judgments, which was evidenced by the formation of the Society for Medical Decision Making, emerging research trends, and the creation of new academic journals. The Society for Medical Decision Making was created after Lee B. Lusted and Eugene L. Saenger organized a conference in Cincinnati, Ohio, in 1979. After this meeting, Lusted and Saenger went on to form the society's first board. Its stated mandate concerned the use of laboratory science in medical decision making. The following year, the society inaugurated its own journal about decision theory, which primarily focused on "newly developed formal approaches to clinical decision making, such as using algorithms and decision tables when investigating common clinical problems" (Flanagin and Lundberg 1990, 279). In the April 1983 issue of the *Journal of the American Medical Association* (*JAMA*), Merz (1983, 2133) describes decision theory, the theory on which the society was founded, as "a systematic approach to decision making under conditions of uncertainty," exploring "probabilistic" versus "categorical" methods, and avoiding "deterministic" understandings of clinical practice. The new focus on probabilities (from Bayesian logic) was intended to replace the taxonomic program suggested by Feinstein.

The goals of the Society for Medical Decision Making opposed the scientificity of laboratory medical science: "Contributing to this distinction is the uncertainty inherent in clinical information, in laboratory test interpretation, in the relationship between clinical findings and disease, and in the effects of treatment" (Merz 1983, 2133). Uncertainty here refers to the subjective interpretation of the results, not the validity of the results themselves. Individual physicians could be flawed in their logic and make poor decisions with poor health outcomes. Further, the remarkable benefits of decision theory, as cited by Merz, were its cost-effective nature and the development of better education practices for training physicians. These two themes continue on in the 1980s and in discussions leading up to EBM.

Statements surfaced purporting and reaffirming the scientific merit of physicians' judgments, arguing that their basis lay in physicians' interpretation of the "facts" collected (King 1983, 2479). Physicians were questioning the incomplete nature of science by appealing to the public mandate of medicine – that it act based on the *best available* knowledge and expertise. Researchers, however, asked questions related to physicians' individual interpretations of evidence. The main cause for concern seemed to be how the knowledge of medical research, such as the results of RCTs, was being used and how this related to questions about risk, treatment, and ethics (Lachlan, Wartman, and Brock 1988, 3166). Because physicians' judgments are subject to "the same errors common to all human cognitive processes" (Silverstein 1988, 1758), these questions led to the development of prediction mechanisms for medical decisions.

The research that was surfacing about variability in the execution of care (e.g., Mulley 1988, 540–41) also seemed to be coming to a turning point. Poor medical judgments came to be associated with clinical practices that were not scientific. Eddy (1990a, 287) describes the changes occurring in medicine that developed from the 1960s through the 1980s as challenges to medical authority:

> What is going on is that one of the basic assumptions under-lying the practice of medicine is being challenged ... Simply put, the assumption is that whatever a physician decides is, by definition, correct. The challenge says that while many decisions no doubt are correct, many are not, and elaborate mechanisms are needed to determine which are which. Physicians are slowly being stripped of their decision-making power.

At about the same time, articles appeared that sought to defend medicine as a public trust in order to improve the health of the population through research, training and education, and patient care (e.g., Schroeder, Zones, and Showstack 1989). The problem was that the public still invested in medicine to provide the best possible care to its members, but the public no longer valued the laboratory as the standard for measuring care. It was becoming evident that the clinician's decisions were not the final authority on the execution of care. Instead, given that the health of the public was entrusted to each individual physician, there was a need to know which decisions were right and which were wrong.

Eddy (1990a, 290) offers the following: "The solution is not to remove the decision-making power from physicians, but to improve the capacity of physicians to make better decisions. To achieve this solution, we must give physicians the information they need; we must institutionalize the skills to use that information; and we must build processes that support, not dictate, decisions." The new science of clinical epidemiology provided a justification for formulating individual decision making and doctor-patient interaction. The use of information or evidence in clinical practice would be institutionalized as one of the programmatic principles of the McMaster medical school, the implications of which I discuss in Chapter 3.

Building on this momentum, in 1988 the *Journal of Clinical Epidemiology* was founded by Feinstein and Walter O. Spitzer (a Canadian). Sackett also served on the first editorial board. In the inaugural issue, Feinstein announced his reasons for changing the name of the journal (formerly the *Journal of Chronic Diseases*) and its new emphasis on an emerging field: "The change of name, however, is merely a new label for the same wine. Everything else remains intact ... The new title simply reflects the principle of 'truth of labelling.' It indicates distinctions that have actually been present in the 'wine' for a long time" (Feinstein and Spitzer 1988, 1). Feinstein notes that, while some researchers may be repelled by the name change during a time when the definition and methods of clinical epidemiology were under debate, he hoped that the journal would help to start a movement to include the methods of clinical epidemiology in all aspects of medical practice (6–7). This name change and new emphasis on the part of an important medical journal points to changes in the field of medicine and the shift to a more scientific approach to clinical practice.

Some physicians argued that the scientific approach to clinical practice was a result of the tension between the art and science of medicine. The research that was surfacing about variability in the execution of care (e.g., Mulley 1988, 540–41) was associated with clinical practices that were not scientific. Clinical epidemiology provided a basis for translating knowledge about statistical probabilities into the bedside care setting. For this reason, the science of medicine was associated with a uniformity of care and a systematized strategy for making clinical judgments on a scientific (i.e., a predictable and reproducible) basis, whereas uncertainty was thought to come from the "art" side of medicine: "The traditional medical response to uncertainty ... comprises a knowledge base derived from the clinician's own individual clinical experience interpreted in the light of the collective experience of the profession, learned through apprenticeship to eminent practitioners, usually in technically sophisticated teaching hospitals" (Daly 2005, 10). The problem was, according to an interview with Kerr White, the "uncritical acceptance of biomedical science as the only scientific basis for evaluating the benefits and risks of clinical practice, and it derived ... from the historical dominance of laboratory science in hospitals" (42). A journal devoted to clinical epidemiology is an index of the shift towards providing a scientific rationale for clinical judgments, and its goal was to resolve the problems of their practice in the institution of medicine across a number of sites of practice.

Linking Practice and Outcomes

Alongside conversations about the decision-making power of physicians, questions emerged about the effects and outcomes of medical education and physician training. One study questioned whether better education programs for physicians actually result in improved patient health (Tosteson 1990, 234–38). Tosteson argues that medical education should give students the skills to self-educate by implementing science as a part of clinical practice. Another example of these questions may be found in an American study that tested 112 physicians. It asked respondents to evaluate the clinical decisions presented in vignette cases, and the results showed mass disagreement between respondents about whether a negative outcome for a patient was a result of inappropriate care (Caplan, Posner, and Cheney 1991, 1960). This study shows that clinical judgments were evaluated based on outcome rather than, say, on the physician's method of reasoning. Further, a massive review of physician education revealed that continuing medical education led to better physician performance (and sometimes better health care outcomes), thus stressing the importance of continued medical education (Davis et al. 1992, 1116).

The many statements that were gathered in the 1980s and into the early 1990s were underpinned by disputes over variations in how clinicians interpreted evidence, provided care for patients with similar illnesses, and evaluated whether the outcome of that care was appropriate or inappropriate. The EBM Working Group appeared in response to these concerns, and it was an attempt to intervene in the debates about clinical practice. The quest for better evidence was not just a solution to the problems of clinical judgment but also a means by which recommendations for reducing or resolving those problems in clinical care could be articulated, justified, and subsequently implemented.

From Clinical Epidemiology to EBM

The problems that culminated in the 1980s concerned: 1) the scientific basis of care, 2) the authority of medicine, 3) the relationship of medicine to the broader public, and 4) the contested nature of the link between physician training and curriculum reform for the improvement of health care. As mentioned, these conversations responded to disputes over variations in the ways that clinicians interpreted evidence, provided care for patients with similar illnesses, and determined that the outcome of care was appropriate or inappropriate. It was out of these concerns that the EBM Working Group appeared, making a "move from a clinical epidemiology located in research to an attempt to intervene in clinical practice" (Mykhalovskiy and Weir 2004, 1065). As I show later on, the quest for better evidence was not just a solution to issues about the problematization of clinical practice but also a means by which recommendations for eliminating or reducing those problems in clinical care could be articulated and subsequently implemented. In this section, I demonstrate the shift in the relations of discourse that gave rise to clinical epidemiology and the emergence of EBM.

The problematization of clinical judgment in the medical literature led to the emergence of new methods of clinical reasoning in the burgeoning science of clinical epidemiology. A number of books in the late 1970s and 1980s appeared in an attempt to help physicians to interpret evidence that could be found in the medical literature. For example, Engelhardt and colleagues' 1977 book, *Clinical Judgment: A Critical Appraisal,* makes a case for reviewing the methods of clinical reasoning taught in medical education training programs; and Sackett and colleagues' 1985 textbook, *Clinical Epidemiology: A Basic Science for Clinical Medicine,* attempts to teach people how to use research in clinical care. These books provided a liberal solution to the problematization of clinical judgment: educate individual clinicians so that they can better bring together science and clinical experience and expertise. A method known as "critical appraisal" was taken up by researchers at McMaster University, and it located the site for institutional interventions in clinical reasoning. Here I provide evidence to support Mykhalovskiy and Weir's (2004, 1065) claim that the "intervention of EBM in clinical reason is an attempt to take the probabilistic rationality resulting from clinical trials and attach it to previously existing forms of clinical knowledge." The following chapter discusses how these solutions were actually installed in institutional education and training programs, but here I spell out the discursive links between clinical epidemiology's articulation of the solutions to the problems to which the discipline responded as well as to EBM as a discursive practice. To do this, I discuss the clinical appraisal method, which is the basis for EBM.

The critical appraisal method is defined as "the application of rules of evidence to clinical and published data in order to determine their own validity and applicability" (Easterbrook 1990,

392). Ideally, this method would be used in clinical practice to determine the value of prescribing diagnostic tests, to understand the validity of statements about the mechanisms of a disease, and to determine the effectiveness of different therapeutic interventions via appraisal of the literature. Before making a clinical decision, the physician would employ this method to examine the medical literature. If a patient presented with certain symptoms, this method could help determine which diagnostic test to order or which therapy to prescribe: reviewing the literature could give the physician a sense of confidence about which tests would provide the most sensitive results or, based on population data, which therapy would be most applicable to this particular patient. This method was to be used for answering a clinical question and would provide some scientificity to clinical decision making. The literature on the clinical appraisal method generally highlights the paucity of statistical analysis in medical education, and it teaches doctors how to peruse the literature so that they might integrate it into their practices even though they lack substantive training in statistics. If physicians were to learn this method, they could resolve the problems associated with clinical care that emerged as a result of advances in technology and scientific research.

The critical appraisal method sought to empower physicians to adjudicate the science for themselves and to better inform their clinical decision making: "The purpose of appraising a paper is to discover if the methods and results of the research are sufficiently valid to produce useful information" (Fowkes and Fulton 1991, 1136). The method focused on paying particular attention to specific questions when reading the medical literature, such as an assessment of the variation in study design between articles about the same therapy. It allowed physicians to understand and highlight the types of risk – and the methods to control for risk – when applying research results to an individual clinical patient. This method proposed to respond to the concerns in the medical literature about the relationship between medical research and the clinic, practice variation, measurement, and clinical authority. Critical appraisal responded to what two physicians called the "need for systematized judgment" (Drachman and Hart 1972, 996).

The method consisted of the following steps: assessing the abstract; identifying the research objectives and the study design; assessing the usefulness of statistical findings and results, including the inclusion criteria, study group selection, and the quality of measurements and outcomes in the study (Fowkes and Fulton 1991, 1136–38). Performing the steps of critical appraisal led to a clinical judgment, which ultimately relied on the expertise of the clinician (1140). There remained a tension between the expertise of the clinician and the systematic nature of the appraisal.

How this method, which emerged at McMaster, gained such traction in the medical literature was a question of exposure and its sensitivity to the pulse of medicine – that is, it targeted prevalent anxieties about problematized uncertainties. The later development and dominance of EBM depended on the success of this method and its formulation of the problems with clinical decision making. In 1981, the *Canadian Medical Association Journal* (*CMAJ*) published an article titled "How to Read Clinical Journals," which was authored by the Department of Clinical Epidemiology and Biostatistics (CE&B) at McMaster University. This article begins by stating the problem facing most clinicians at the time, which was that they should be spending more time reading medical literature. But this is nearly impossible: "To keep up with the 10 leading journals in internal medicine a clinician must read 200 articles and 70 editorials per month" (CE&B 1981, 555). The problem of there being too much information for clinicians to use as evidence in their practices could be resolved through CE&B's recommendations regarding how clinicians ought to read medical journals, which, if employed correctly, could produce greater efficiency in practice due to an ability to assess the validity and applicability of medical literature.

The article provides a case study of hypertension in health care in Hamilton, Ontario, which found that the physician's decision to treat and manage the condition could be correlated with the year that physician graduated from medical school. There was ongoing practice variation: "It appeared that these physicians, both older and younger, were practicing the sort of medicine that prevailed at the time they finished their training. They had been taught the appropriate contemporaneous management of hypertension but often appeared not to have been taught how to decide when to change this management" (CE&B 1981, 555). These findings served to justify the need to change therapeutic strategies and decision making; as a physician's career progresses, the best information changes, which makes it difficult to make decisions that are consistent with best evidence in the medical literature. Being "behind in reading" meant that the clinician was "falling short" in clinical practice (556). The authors stated that there was more than just a need for continuing medical education, which was already a licensing requirement in Canada. Physicians needed to have better reading skills: clinicians shouldn't read any journal article as the authority on what to do or how to treat patients; rather, they should read the available literature and decide for themselves if the study would be useful to their presenting patient(s) (557). The ultimate concern with reading the article or literature was applicability: physicians needed to learn how to apply evidence in their practice with a discerning eye. The article concludes by noting that good reading could also be cost-effective (the physician would not order unnecessary tests or prescribe ineffective therapies) (558).

In this CE&B article, one may observe the problematization of practice variation and the individual interpretation of evidence. The solution the authors propose not only targets the physician's reading skills but also stipulates that these skills could be improved to resolve the issues with clinical reasoning. Medical authority is also under question as the article contends that physicians should not trust the authority of medical journals: "Review and editorial policies of even the best and most highly respected journals provide incomplete protection from error, and a single subscription can provide both truth and a carnival of bias" (CE&B 1981, 558). Learning how to read the literature and appraise it should form the basis of the authority of clinical judgments. In the same year, CE&B (1981) published an article in the *Canadian Medical Association Journal (CMAJ)* titled "How to Read Clinical Journals, I: Why Read Them and How to Start Reading Them Critically." This article became the most requested reprint from *CMAJ* (Guyatt and Rennie 1993, 2096). In 1993, its popularity would spur a series on how to read and apply evidence in clinical practice. Members of CE&B also published two editions of a textbook titled *Clinical Epidemiology: A Basic Science for Clinical Medicine,* which deals with the same subject matter and also indicates the traction that the critical appraisal method was gaining among practitioners and educators.

The McMaster CE&B program later provided data to support the use of its method. In 1987, CE&B researchers published "Controlled Trial of Teaching Critical Appraisal to Medical Students," which uses the highest form of evidence in the EBM hierarchy to measure the impact of a curricular innovation in medical training (Bennett et al. 1987, 2451–54). They define the critical appraisal method as follows:

Critical appraisal comprises the ability to assess the validity and applicability of clinical, paraclinical, and published evidence and to incorporate the results of this assessment into patient management. It is based on the premise that to be effective in maintaining or improving the health of their patients, clinicians must base the care they give on sound scientific evidence that it does more good than harm. (2451)

Their justification for using the critical appraisal method builds on the earlier publication regarding the importance of reading the medical literature and applying useful evidence in practice. They conclude that clinical appraisal training allowed clerks and tutors to excel on exams pertaining to the use of diagnostic tests (37 percent better than the control group, which received no training) and therapeutic interventions (8 percent better than the control group) (2451). The article also responds to the problematized authority of medical research, indicating that, because students of medical science took that authority for granted, they did not know how to assess the quality of science used in the clinic. The authors propose to resolve this issue by showing that their study enables them to test the interventions of their unique curriculum (2455). The members of the control group of students were not taught the critical appraisal method, and they seemed more likely to accept the authority of the medical literature than did those trained under the new curriculum. Bennett and colleagues argue that their study serves as evidence to justify making a change to the medical curriculum at McMaster: "Clerkship planning committee, and later its parent medical education committee, [will] add critical appraisal skills to clinical skills and self-directed learning skills as fundamental objectives of McMaster University's undergraduate MD program" (2454). I discuss the changes to the medical school at McMaster in detail in the next two chapters, where I move from establishing the relations of discourse that connected the emergence of clinical epidemiology to EBM to focusing on the conditions that allowed these methods to become dominant in social space.

The appearance of critical appraisal in two international journals of medicine serves as my final example of the link between the problematization of clinical practice and the emergence of EBM. First, in 1991 Gordon Guyatt (one of the members of EBM Working Group) published an article in *ACP Journal Club*. The article begins with a vignette that focuses on a physician who wants to understand the diagnostic properties of a test, its sensitivity and specificity, and wants to understand how to search the literature and apply this knowledge to an individual patient. Here, for the first time, the method of critical appraisal and EBM are brought together: "For the clinician, evidence-based medicine requires skills of literature retrieval, critical appraisal, and information synthesis" (Guyatt 1991, A16). The term "evidence-based medicine" would come to replace the term "critical appraisal method." Guyatt makes clear the importance of critical appraisal in improving the future of medicine:

The way of the future described above depicts an important advance in the inclusion of new evidence into clinical practice. Clinicians were formerly taught to look to authority (whether a textbook, an expert lecturer, or a local senior physician) to resolve issues of patient management. Evidence-based medicine uses additional strategies, including quickly tracking down publications of studies that are directly relevant to the clinical problem, critically appraising these studies, and applying the results of the best studies to the clinical problem at hand. (A16)

Guyatt indicates that the thematic concerns with medical authority and the use of research in clinical decision making were resolved by learning to read the literature. Compare the above quotation to the first statements pertaining to EBM, where the EBM Working Group describes it as follows: "EBM requires new skills of the physician, including efficient literature searching and the application of formal rules of evidence evaluating the clinical literature" (Guyatt et al. 1992, 2420). EBM was an effort to codify, in medical discourse, the problems of medical practice and to intervene at the level of individual judgments. It involved the clinician's ability to read and evaluate medical research in order to apply it properly to their patients.

In the year following the first utterances of EBM, the *Journal of the American Medical Association* launched its Users' Guides to the Medical Literature series. McMaster clinician-researchers, who were also members of the EBM Working Group, began this series in an attempt to instruct physicians across the world in how to keep up with the fast-paced world of medicine. Guyatt's introduction to the series of articles states that the series is a reply to the following question: "How can physicians learn about new information and innovations, and decide how (if at all) they should modify their practice?" (Guyatt and Rennie 1993, 2096). Later statements explain the rationale for the series: "Our clinical journals are abound with reports documenting inexcusable delays and inexplicable variations in the incorporation of evidence into traditional medical practice, sometimes even in the same institutions in which the primary evidence was generated" (White et al. 1995, 840). At the time of this writing, the series is ongoing and has been recently revived, demonstrating an ongoing endorsement of EBM and the attempts to ameliorate its application to practice.

The *JAMA* series not only provided exposure to the term "evidence-based medicine" but also played a role in proliferating the problematization of clinical judgment associated with physician reasoning. There was an increase in the number of statements about the applicability of research to practice, and the introductory article serves as an example of the synthetic work involved in bringing all the problems with clinical judgment into one arena, where the methods of EBM can offer a solution. For example, the article notes the problems with medical authority: "[Clinicians] may choose to believe the most authoritative expert or the trusted colleague, but they have difficulty exercising independent judgment" (Guyatt and Rennie 1993, 2096). The article advances the assumption that new information produced by scientific research should modify clinical practice, which is reminiscent of earlier concerns regarding the relevance of the laboratory to bedside care and to which clinical epidemiology responded. The *JAMA* series is about the "need for an even more intense focus on using the medical literature to solve real patient problems," and this focus is referred to as EBM (ibid.). Not only did the article state that the use of evidence gleaned from "systematic overview, practice guidelines, decision analysis and economic analysis" could improve patient care but also that "optimal patient care in the 1990s requires an ability to use the medical literature to solve clinical problems" (2096–97). The purpose of the series was to empower physicians who wanted to become more "quantitative" in their thinking about clinical decision making by emphasizing to them the importance of relevance and validity.

Clinical epidemiology and its solutions to the problematization of various elements of clinical practice served as the discursive precondition for the appearance of the term "evidence-based medicine" and its dominant status in the medical discourse. EBM was the proposed solution to the culmination of a series of ongoing concerns, new measurements, and new solutions – the physician could be trained to better interpret, integrate, and apply useful evidence in her practice in order to eliminate the identified problems of medical practice. Critical appraisal, a method whose objective was to ameliorate the reading skills of clinicians, located the site for intervention in the physician's judgment. Research studies concerning the use of evidence in practice – that is, the use of the critical appraisal method – founded a program and curriculum whose purpose was to achieve better physician training. The rationale for the importance of the critical appraisal method refers to the problem of the physician's relationship to the literature as, in the words of social scientist Eric Mykhalovskiy, "ambivalent." In his research on "ambivalent reading," Mykhalovskiy examines ongoing efforts in the 1990s to encourage physician reading of medical literature. He analyzes data from *Informed,* a newsletter for family physicians. His investigations focus on how texts govern productively through the freedom of the physician's judgment, pointing out that EBM governs physicians as "indifferent readers" (Mykhalovskiy 2003, 331). This being the case, physicians need to be encouraged and taught how to read better through focusing on "how and what they read": "Evidence ... is produced with the intention of being entered into physicians' clinical activities" (332). While his research draws on Dorothy Smith's (1990) notion of texts as "relations of ruling," my genealogical research furthers his conclusions by exploring how the discursive practice of reading targets the clinician's judgment.

Dominant Prescriptions: Repetition in Medical Problems

Evidence-based medicine has not been without its critics. In this section I document the challenges to the EBM model of decision making and show how it has responded. In EBM, the assumptions that underlie the problematization of clinical judgment have led to the repetition of the same problems: the solutions that were and continue to be proposed in the relations of discourse simply generate the same sorts of issues. In other words, the discursive field of EBM reintroduces the same problems of measurement, authority, and practice variation that it had initially aimed to resolve.[7]

After the initial appearance of EBM, practitioners began to ask for a way of assessing evidence in light of there being so much of it. For example, search engines such as MEDLINE, PubMed, and DynaMed provide individual physicians with access to a vast number of medical studies and online tools that help them locate evidence to use in their clinical practice. In the early 1990s, the proliferation of computer and database technology in medicine provided (almost) unlimited resources for clinicians to search out the results of RCTs. According to Straus and Sackett (1998, 318), EBM is considered the best way to keep up with fast-changing information in the medical literature because it applies the most recent and best clinical evidence to practice. New journals have emerged to explicitly manage problems concerning physician time constraints and mass information. These journals translate research evidence from thousands of journals into "answers" to clinical questions by providing recommendations for treatment programs (Davidoff et al. 1995). For example, the *Journal of Evidence-Based Medicine* states: "You'd have to read 227 articles in the *Lancet* or 118 articles in the *New England Journal of Medicine* to get the relevant information that would be contained in 1 Evidence-Based Medicine article" (BMJ Publishing 2013).[8] While this new journal was initially controversial, its creation received accolades from the medical community:

> Although in an ideal world, it might be desirable for every clinician to be equipped, both cognitively and technically, to conduct his own literature searches to find the best evidence to address clinical questions, such a goal is unrealistic, or at best inefficient. It is far more sensible to devise strategies such as *Evidence Based Medicine* has, to help busy clinicians. (Norman and Blau 1995, 1300)

These new journals exist because the doctor, under the EBM program, is required to treat patients based on the best available evidence; this is an onerous task, however, as there is too much information available. *Evidence-Based Medicine* and other tools aim to synthesize research evidence and thus to resolve this problem. Other researchers hypothesized that the increase in available information was affecting physician decision making. Too much information could make it more difficult to make good judgments, leading to error (Redelmeier and Shafir 1995, 302–5).

The Cochrane database also focuses on improving the physician's capacity to make better judgments. The database became an open access library for practising physicians and was referred to as "Britain's gift" to the world (Smith and Chalmers 2001). The database, following EBM, came to be organized by clinical questions: once a physician could formulate a question, which, ideally, she would learn to do in medical school, she would have access to a vast amount of electronic information that could be searched from anywhere. And, since articles in the database synthesized vast amounts of research, this would cut down on the time constraints of clinical practice. Chalmers, Hedges, and Cooper (2002) saw the potential of digital databases both to reduce unequal access to the best clinical information worldwide and to keep "up to date" with the vast amounts of evidence being published daily. The database was a shift from individualized to aggregated evidence, from clinical epidemiology to EBM.

Additionally, concerns about keeping up with this vast amount of information culminated in a series of conversations in the medical literature regarding "practice guidelines," which Eddy (1990b, 3077) defines as "generic decisions – recommendations intended for a collection of patients rather than for a single patient." Practice guidelines were intended to provide a way to determine the "correct" way to provide care. The use of medical evidence, in the form of RCTs, provided a scientific justification for formulating the "art" of decision making and the interpretation of the doctor-patient interaction into a systematic set of procedures.

Original members of the EBM Working Group later endorsed clinical practice guidelines, which they defined as strategies "for changing clinician behaviour: systematically developed statements or recommendations to assist practitioner and patient decisions about appropriate health care for specific clinical circumstances" (Guyatt, Haynes, et al. 2008, 270), Guidelines came to be created through collaborative partnerships between various stakeholders in health care. They assessed evidence through the critical appraisal method in order both to reduce the "guesswork" of medicine, providing a systematic framework for the interpretation of evidence (Sackett et al. 2000, 135–40), and to regulate the assessment of risk (Guyatt, Haynes, et al. 2008, 14). With thousands of guidelines circulating in Canada, the United States, the United Kingdom, and beyond, there were demands to come up with rules for measuring their quality.

AGREE: Meta Standards for Measuring the Quality of Evidence

In 1998, a funding initiative in the European Union formed a collaboration whose goal was to create a "generic instrument that can be used to appraise the quality of clinical guidelines" and to facilitate their development among collaborating countries. The group created the AGREE instrument, which responded to what it saw as a need to assess the quality of evidence used in the dissemination of best practices: "The number of published guidelines proliferates, there have been calls for the establishment of internationally recognized standards to improve the development and reporting of clinical guidelines" (AGREE Collaboration 2003, 18). Some critics have referred to the proliferation of guidelines as "cookbook medicine," whereby doctors are given "recipes" for treating and interacting with patients. These criticisms point to a reappearance of the problem of medical authority: there is a tension in the relations of discourse between best practices as standards for controlling what physicians do, on the one hand, and evidence-based guidelines as allowing individual clinicians to be empowered to make their own judgments, on the other.

In 2002, the Guidelines International Network (GIN) was created as a collaboration among various member groups. Its objective was to let each country, each medical society, decide which guidelines it would endorse. Each society or college could evaluate and research all available guidelines, and, if those guidelines used the AGREE agreement, the society/college would know that they were of high quality. AGREE is an instrument, a rule, a meta-standard used to assess and grade various guidelines and how they use evidence. Sociologist Loes Knaapen (2014, 820) refers to these instruments as "meta-standards called 'guidelines for guidelines.'" These universal standards ensure that local applications of guidelines are using the highest quality evidence and recommendations. The instrument, however, introduces the importance of norms and values as co-determining parts of guideline development and implementation (Knaapen 2013, 79). AGREE allows various nations to select which guidelines they will endorse, given the evidence and the context of the practice setting. If guidelines are meant to standardize practice across geographical contexts, there is potential for the emergence of new forms and variations of practice. In Canada, variation continues as it is up to the provincial medical colleges to endorse the guidelines they choose – and many colleges support different guidelines. Even if guidelines are supported by rigorous standards for evidence through a multiplicity of courses of action, thus thwarting concerns about "cookbook" criticisms (e.g., Berg 1995), various societies support different guidelines, and practices between physicians or regional differences between provinces could be an ongoing issue in medical practice.

Patient Values and EBM

The EBM model continues to be criticized for its lack of patient-centredness. It was suggested in the 1990s that patient experience could be used to measure the "outcome" of a treatment and could improve patient care. Patient experience would be a measure similar to the subjective evaluation of one's satisfaction with medical services. This suggestion, however, was marginalized by the "incorporation of patient values" into EBM; nonetheless, it represents a criticism of the EBM program (Reiser 1993, 1012–17). In EBM, patient values are evidence that factor into a physician's decision. Some researchers call for an increase in the patient's role in health care. For example, one review article details how law, medical decision-making theories, and education are being changed by the movement to include patient values and preferences as "evidence" for making medical judgments (Laine and Davidoff 1996).

Other initiatives to include patients in the practice of EBM include the patient-centred movement. Patient-centred care (PCC) is defined as "the need for clinicians, staff, and health care systems to shift focus away from diseases and back to the patient and family" (Barry and Edgman-Levitan 2012, 780). Various attempts have been made to synthesize the values of medicine with the values of the patient and their family. Evidence-based patient-centred care is defined as "the use of evidence-based information as a way of enhancing people's choices when those people are patients" (Elwyn and Edwards 2009, 7). The concern in the PCC literature, however, is that, under EBM, evidence can be at odds with patient experience and values because the latter are difficult to quantify (Cronje and Fullan 2003, 357–58). Under EBM, physicians are expected to use their clinical expertise to integrate the best evidence, but critics have shown that not only is there a tension between the evidence and evidence-based clinical expertise (e.g., Greenhalgh 1999, 323) but that "the status of scientific data as evidence rests not only in the research itself, but in the diverse communities of physicians who interpret and use them" (Berkwits 1998, 1542). Under EBM, there is a conflict between patient autonomy and the doctor's need to make good judgments (Godolphin 2009, e188).

The PCC approach attempts to overcome these criticisms. The core principle that guides PCC is shared decision making (SDM), whereby "both parties share information: the clinician offers options and describes their risks and benefits, and the patient expresses his or her preferences and values" (Barry and

Edgman-Levitan 2012, 781). SDM allows each to learn from the other and facilitates shared responsibility in any decision about how to proceed. In the literature, SDM is primarily focused on the creation of decision-aids for physicians to share with their patients. These aids come in a variety of formats, including electronic (e.g., Agoritsas et al. 2015), and their purpose is to provide patients with information that will help them make decisions that are consistent with their values, that are based on medical knowledge and perception of risk, and that will enable them to reduce ambivalences and to become more involved in their own care (Barry and Edgman-Levitan 2012, 781). Research in the social sciences has helped improve SDM models (e.g., Satterfield et al. 2009). If PCC and EBM combine, there can be a conscientious and judicious search for choices that "respond to patient's ideas, concerns and expectations" (Godolphin 2009, e187).

Patient preferences and values, however, resist the logic of the EBM hierarchy of evidence. The expert/lay divide between physicians, who have a deep clinical understanding of EBM, and the patients who are intended to use decision-aids to make their decisions remains a target of criticism from both bioethicists and social scientists: "EBM creates a decision-making context in which patients merely select their preferences from a predetermined list of outcomes, rather than helping patients to engage in meaningful reflection" (Bluhm 2009, 135). The literature identifies the role of physician authority in the clinic as an ongoing problem.

To respond to these issues, EBM has made efforts to find a measurement for assessing the incorporation of patient values into medical care. Trends that involve the use of outcomes measurement in order to formulate interventions for the improvement of care continued throughout the 1990s. These initiatives were formulated on the premise that evidence-based changes lead to good recommendations. Debates about the role of quality of life measures were also gaining momentum; these measures were the standard by which the outcome of medical judgments could be measured. For example, Leplège and Hunt (1997) asked how medicine ought to measure quality of life in order to quantify such a "subjective" category. Their article follows up on an article by Guyatt and colleagues (1989, 1447) that reviews and recommends a variety of scientific instruments for measuring quality of life so as to more effectively determine the outcomes of RCTs. Leplège and Hunt aimed to give scientific, objective validity to patient experiences so as to include a patient-centred measurement in the execution of evidence-based medical practice. If EBM could measure quality of life (something that patients typically valued), they could rank evidence in light of these issues. However, PCC, being a largely "subjective" or "preferential" indicator, is difficult to determine under the principles of EBM. There are conflicts between the objectives of PCC and those of EBM. What ought to be done, and on what basis – the authority of medicine or the patient's needs – may not readily be rendered intelligible by EBM. And these concerns continue to resurface in the medical discourse.

For example, on August 3, 2012, in a *Sunrise Rounds* blog post titled "Against Medical Advice?," Doctor James Salwitz, an oncologist, wrote about a difficult decision: a patient was faced with the choice of whether to have an operation that would require him to use a colostomy bag for the rest of his life but that would almost certainly, according to the evidence, prolong his life significantly. The patient chose not to have the operation, which increased his chances of the cancer returning. Salwitz writes about the difficulty of supporting a patient's decision that goes against the evidence: "Stan's choice is not supported by research, data, my personal experience, nor by experts in the field. Nonetheless, if he decides to choose that path [decline the operation], I will support him" (Salwitz 2012). The necessity to use the best evidence, which EBM requires, means that any judgment against that evidence, even if it is in the patient's best interests, is not necessarily evidence-based, and this revives concerns about the basis of clinical decision making: Are decisions sometimes based on the physician's *subjective* understanding? Other critics of EBM have upheld the need for good evidence: "The definition of evidence is important ... because it illustrates the struggle between patients, scientists, doctors, and public health administrators over the interpretation of scientific results and how to decide the proper goals of medicine" (Saarni and Gylling 2004, 172). The discourse of EBM aims to incorporate patient values into its logic as a form of evidence, but this reproduces problematizations regarding the basis of clinical judgment and, subsequently, regarding what the physician ought to do.

The Changing World: Social and Material Constraints

Within the relations of EBM discourse there are also problems that become relevant as a result of events external to medicine: the discipline and practice needed to adapt to a changing world. For example, physicians often noted generational shifts between incoming cohorts of students. The students of the 1960s and 1970s, for example, were attuned to the civil rights movements happening in North America and beyond, and they wanted to practise medicine in a way that recognized the shifting landscape of power, of inclusion and exclusion. For this reason, medical education, its training and practice, needed to follow suit. Further, the success of the Cochrane database was due, in part, to its embrace of emerging electronic technologies: it did not depend on journal space, where word count and paper and pages determined what and how evidence could be published (e.g., Starr et al. 2009). The institution of medicine produces knowledge within the context of various social constraints, which raises ongoing questions about the capacity for evidence-based practice to reduce subjective or moral judgments or other biases.

Another recent concern in the literature has to do with the status of medical knowledge in relation to funding research. There are many concerns about the role of commercial interests and stakeholders in the EBM literature: To what extent can research produce good evidence if it has been co-opted by capitalist interests? Bioethicists, doctors, and social scientists (e.g., Cooper and Waldby 2014; Matheson 2008) have raised concerns about the pharmaceutical industry's husbandry of EBM. The problem is fundamental to EBM, however, as the highest forms of evidence – RCTs and meta-analyses of RCTs – require large investments in order to carry out the development and multiphasic testing of would-be approved treatments. Private industry has contributed to the production of evidence because patenting the next big thing, like tamoxifen or Viagra,[9] could be worth billions of dollars in revenue. Alarms have sounded about what role a profit motive might play in the production of scientific evidence. How could EBM exist without those large studies of population-based research?

Patient groups are also playing an increasing role in generating new directions in research initiatives and health policy. In Canada, for example, when the Zamboni treatment appeared in the medical literature regarding a possible cure for multiple sclerosis symptoms, it was met with criticism from the medical community but with interest from patient groups. The Multiple Sclerosis Society of Canada was successful in securing national funding from the Canadian Institutes of Health Research for a task force to investigate and test the claims of the Zamboni hypothesis and the "liberation treatment." As Carlos Novas's (2006, 302) research shows, patient groups play a significant role in influencing the production of medical research and guidelines: "Through working alongside scientists, health professionals and political authorities, they [patient groups] attempt to shape in the present the future health and well-being of specific populations." Campaigning on the part of disease-specific patient organizations can influence the production of medical knowledge in accordance with the values of those patients whom the condition affects. The conditions of knowledge production raise concerns in the medical literature about evidence: Can medical knowledge be produced on a scientific basis without being hijacked by the interests of some specific group (is it, for example, associated with commercial industry or patients?). While EBM has tried to address these issues, they continue to surface. The dynamic involvement of interested stakeholders influences the way that funding to pursue scientific research in disease classification and treatment effectiveness is generated.

Conclusion

The various problems identified in the literature rendered medical judgments "amenable to intervention" (Osborne, Rose, and Savage 2008, 521). The emergence of EBM depended on a set of problems that had been identified in the field of clinical practice: the relationship between the laboratory and everyday clinical interactions; the authority of the doctor's decisions; and whether or not physicians keep abreast of the rapidly changing technology and information about disease, the body, and treatments. These problems reveal a disjuncture between what science can measure and what can be known in the clinical setting, and they led to an impetus to justify what goes on in clinical practice. The institution of medicine responded to them by establishing relations of discourse that provide the rules for formulating a scientific basis for systematic clinical judgment: the results of medical research could be translated into recommendations for clinical practice and education reform. The emergence of clinical epidemiology was an attempt to merge the scientific foundations of biomedicine and biometric statistics with the clinical judgments made by individual doctors. Also, the creation of new medical databases provided the "evidence" necessary for bringing scientific knowledge into clinical practice at a time when there was so much uncertainty about the hasty embrace of new technologies and the inability to keep up to date with the best information for making diagnoses and offering treatment. The first glimmerings of EBM appeared on a discursive terrain that had targeted the problematic character of individual judgments.

The problematization of clinical judgment in the field of medicine generated new methods of thinking that, in turn, generated new lines of action. Intervening at the level of the individual clinician's judgment became the juridical solution to certain identified problems. EBM was not necessarily a "new" paradigm, as was initially claimed; rather, it was the manifestation of bringing the emerging science of clinical epidemiology to the bedside. These practices and procedures rendered the problem of medical judgments "visible" (Osborne and Rose 1997, 98) – that is, it rendered them the object of a new science that claimed to improve medical practice. As I explain in the next chapter, these problematizations led to the formulation of the scientific basis by which programs for intervening could be proposed and implemented. Individual expertise would be replaced by knowledge produced by medical research. Rearticulating the problems identified within the clinic in scientific terms rendered medical judgments amenable to scientific measurement and regulation. These interventions in clinical practice then produced the possibility for further intervention. Now that I have discussed the dominant relations of discourse that rendered clinical judgment intelligible and "scientific," I shift my focus to the material conditions that came to organize human activity.

2

Institutional Sites: McMaster University and Canada's Contribution to Medical Training

HAVING JUST EXPLORED the questions emerging in medicine from the 1960s onward, I now consider some of the social conditions that allowed clinical epidemiology and (later) evidence-based medicine to become the dominant relations of discourse and their implications for medical research and teaching. How did these relations of discourse take form? In what institutions? And under what social circumstances? I make explicit the links between various problematizations of medical practice (established in an order of discourse) and the material and spatial relations that would come to reorganize medical activity. By showing how clinical epidemiology was an antecedent of what would later be reformulated as evidence-based medicine, I explain how institutional, political, and economic relations supported a particular way of speaking about the problems of medical care and how the solution that clinical epidemiology offered to this problem became dominant in Western medical practice.

In a historical case study of Ontario's McMaster University, where the first department of clinical epidemiology was created, I explain how the relations of discourse came to be institutionalized. This department preceded the first statements of EBM, and it was at McMaster that the EBM approach to medical training and practice was first institutionalized. By examining institutional structures, I was able see how the new science of clinical epidemiology was, to paraphrase Foucault (1980b, 146), "effectively inscribed in social space." The new way of articulating and intervening in

clinical judgment required a new form of curriculum and organization of space, which, again following Foucault, I argue "was at
once the effect and the support" (146) for the emerging program
of conduct. By analyzing the conditions that led to the establishment of a new training program and hospital, I show the workings
of the relations of power (149) and the role they played in stabiliz-
ing the scientific discourse of clinical epidemiology in medicine.

Medical Education at McMaster University: Funding and Institutional Support

This section first explores the political landscape within which
the medical curriculum of the 1960s was considered out of date. I
discuss how reports and funding from the provincial government
enabled the creation of the McMaster medical school. It began
with the Ontario Ministry of Education, which was under increasing "pressure from the ... College of Physicians and Surgeons of
Ontario to bring to the attention of Government the urgent need
for a new ... Faculty of Medicine."[1]

Although the creation of McMaster's medical school took place
over a few years in the latter half of the 1960s, the location of a
new medical school had been a topic of discussion between the
president of McMaster and the minister of education since 1956.[2]
Five years later, H.G. Thode, then vice-president and director of
research, wrote a report to Premier Robarts titled "McMaster University and Medical Education."[3] This document cited the results
from a visit to the McMaster campus by Sir Francis Fraser, and
it summarized plans for the opening of a new medical school at
McMaster, "if and when an additional medical school is needed in
Ontario" (1).

Ontario education is regulated and funded by the provincial
government. At the time (the early 1960s), there was no special
ministry responsible for universities and colleges. Instead, the
Department of University Affairs was a subcommittee of, and
reported to, Ontario's minister of education. The Committee on
University Affairs was created by the Department of University

Affairs Act in 1964 (OC 4157/64) to respond to increasing enrolments and new program needs in Ontario's universities. The committee had a primary goal: "To study matters concerning the establishment, development, operation, expansion and financing of universities in Ontario and to make recommendations thereon to the Minister of University Affairs for the information and advice of the Government" (OC 4157/64, subsection 3.3). This committee was in charge of liaising with Ontario universities for the purpose of making recommendations about new programs and improvements to the Ministry of Education.

Simultaneously, in 1964 the Royal Commission on Health Services published its first report. The commission's task was to

> inquire into and report upon the existing facilities and the future need for health services for the people of Canada and the resources to provide such services, and to recommend such measures, consistent with the constitutional division of legislative powers in Canada, as the Commissioners believe will ensure that the best possible health care is available to all Canadians. (Health Canada 2004)

This report was widely considered to be a scathing review of Canadian Health Services. Among the recommendations in the 1964 report, thirty-six pertained directly to universities and three dealt explicitly with Canadian medical programs in Ontario. In order to remedy many of the identified problems, the report recommended the creation of two new medical schools in Ontario. McMaster University was explicitly named as the site of one of the new schools. The report also suggested that the federal and provincial governments should make equal financial commitments to the new schools.

Following the release of the report in 1964, John P. Robarts, premier of Ontario, approved plans for the development of the McMaster medical school. Subsequently, he announced the expansion of the teaching facilities for medicine at McMaster. In a 1966 report created by McMaster University for the Committee on University Affairs, the findings from the Royal Commission on Health Services were cited as a rationale for the creation of a new approach "to the education of health personnel and to develop more effective ways of utilizing staff and facilities."[4] The report recommended that new approaches to medical education ought to be undertaken because Ontario's current medical school programs were out of date: "The evidence that our present schools of medicine required extensive renovation and expansion to bring them up to standards acceptable for our times is overwhelming."[5] There was also new interest in creating a "health sciences centre" to house hospital activities, clinical research activities, and instruction. The McMaster medical school would be built on the assumption that the current methods of medical training and practice were insufficient. The support for the new program at McMaster is evidenced by the allocation of provincial grants totalling $50 million [$405 million][6] during 1965–66.[7]

The ideas contained within the Royal Commission on Health Services can be found in other published reports from the 1960s. They emphasized increasing the role that university education would play in medical training and insisted that enrolments in the health sciences should meet the demands and needs of society. A report titled "From the Sixties to the Seventies: An Appraisal of Higher Education in Ontario by the Presidents' Research Committee for the Committee of Presidents of Universities of Ontario" (1966) was prepared for the Honourable John P. Robarts, minister of education for Ontario. In it H.G. Thode, then president of McMaster, wrote about the plans for the location of the new medical school; he included information about the resources needed to open the medical school as well as the schedule for its preparations, courses, and construction. He hoped that the first class at McMaster would begin in 1967.[8] His report proposed a new model of medical training. There were three major differences between the old model and the new model: 1) hiring full-time clinical training staff (that was previously part-time), 2) increasing the role of research in medical training and practice, and 3) establishing a university hospital on the McMaster campus. In the following subsection, I show how the justification for the creation of the first clinical epidemiology department, and its role in the medical program more generally, was a response to the various problematizations of clinical judgment.

Putting It All Together: Creating a Medical Program for Researchers and Clinicians

After Ontario approved the new medical program, President Thode appointed John Evans as the dean of medicine to coordinate the development of the program and to appoint faculty members to its new departments. Evans hired David Sackett, a physician and clinical epidemiologist who was in the early part of his career. Sackett's views on the relationship between research and clinical care were shaped by the rising concerns detailed in the previous chapter. He would help create a new curriculum for McMaster University, which would become known for its innovative approach to medical practice.

In a document about his reflections on the history of McMaster's medical program, John Evans wrote:

> At the time, we recognized several problems of high priority related to the practice of medicine in Canada. That too few physicians were being trained was evident from the shortage of Canadian physicians and the yearly licensure of physicians of whom a large percentage were foreign-trained. In Canada ... health professionals were poorly integrated in the care of many patients and had potential skills which were not fully utilized. Nevertheless, the cost of medical care in Canada was rising rapidly.[9]

The program for the new McMaster medical school would offer a solution to these problems, which were also manifesting themselves in the literature (and government documents) about the effectiveness of medical care and were being variously

identified by practitioners and the public alike. Evans item-
ized a number of problems particular to medical schools: 1) the
separation between the university and the medical college; 2)
the isolated and individualized nature of medical practice after
graduation and licensing; 3) the ignorance of individual doctors
about the systemic issues that affected the delivery and organization of their care; and 4) the lack of ongoing education of
physicians after graduation, when they too often failed to "keep
abreast of the ever-changing scientific background to medical
practice."[10]

The objectives of the medical program were crafted so as to
address those problems. In the early statements for the creation
of the MD program, Evans included the following objectives: 1)
the importance for graduates to be able to "identify and define
health problems, and search for information to resolve or manage these problems"; 2) develop "the clinical skills and methods
required to define and manage the health problems of patients";
3) "become a self-directed learner, recognizing personal educational needs, selecting appropriate learning resources, and
evaluating progress"; and 4) "assess professional activity, both
personal and that of other health professionals."[11] The problematization of the disjuncture between the laboratory and the clinic
could be resolved by training new physicians to use the information attained from reading medical journals and applying
the results of these studies directly in their practices. Students
should be relying on scientific evidence in their clinical decision
making, while also keeping up with the latest knowledge and
discoveries.

Making the translation from the results of medical research
to the bedside would require that students know how to apply
population-based data to individual patients. The first clinical epidemiology and biostatistics department in Western medicine was
created to meet this demand in the Faculty of Medicine at McMaster. Despite being a relatively new field for research, CE&B would
come to greatly influence the McMaster curriculum. Sackett was
appointed as the first chairman of CE&B in December 1967.[12] The

McMaster Senate ratified the creation of CE&B on January 10, 1968, with the following statement:

> In the field of medicine, it is becoming increasingly apparent that the identification of causal mechanisms of disease occurrence, the elucidation of the natural history of health and disease, and the planning and evaluation of programmes of therapeutic and preventive measures requires the fusion of traditional methodologies from both clinical medicine and epidemiology. Although the applicability of epidemiologic and biostatistical techniques to problems of clinical and laboratory research is acknowledged, these latter disciplines do not, at present, include advanced competency in the former areas in their training programs. It is proposed, therefore, that an appropriate focus of competency in clinically oriented epidemiology and biostatistics be established at a Departmental level, in the Faculty of Medicine of McMaster University.[13]

The department was created to facilitate collaboration between research and clinical practice at both regional and educational program training levels. These goals were formed on the basis of expertise that would expand beyond the concerns of clinical epidemiology or biostatistics alone. The department noted that, among a number of applications, its role included health economics and health policy analysis.[14]

The medical program would hire full-time clinical staff to teach in the university, which was an improvement over the previous model, which hired part-time staff. This new approach would come to change the operation of medical education by affecting university budgeting, as evidenced in the 1968 "Report of the Committee on University Affairs" created by the Committee on University Affairs (Douglas T. Wright Chairman):

> These changes, the rapidly increasing commitment to medical research, and the very high salaries required to compete with the opportunities offered by private medical practice, make the

cost implication for the future quite staggering ... While much more work will be required, there is already indication that the total cost of operation of medical faculties of the future, with their extra-ordinarily heavy commitment to research and their direct involvement in providing health care, cannot be seen simply as the cost of medical education, but must be acknowledged and supported as part of the total commitment by society to the development of health services.[15]

The funding structure for medical programs was also changing, enabling the marriage between academic research and clinical training, and the justifications for this were founded on the need to integrate research with the clinic.

The problematization of the link between medical science and its application to clinical practice can also be observed in the CE&B's purpose for contributing to the medical program. In the first prospectus that Sackett wrote for the Faculty of Medicine at McMaster in 1967, he proposed that the creation of the CE&B department was necessary in order to facilitate the introduction of the new medical curriculum. He referred to a new approach, called the "critical incident" approach,[16] which was to focus on teaching "statistics without numbers" so that the "practical application" of clinical epidemiology could be implemented in the care of individual patients.[17]

In 1972, CE&B placed the emphasis on the relationship between medical research and its utilization in practice.[18] In "Objectives: Department of Clinical Epidemiology and Biostatistics," a document that was created following the approval of the department prospectus and the proposal for the curriculum of study, CE&B articulated the department as a kind of under-labourer for methodology in collaboration with the research needs of the other departments in the Faculty of Medicine. CE&B "must strive to develop learning resources relevant to the practice of medicine ... [and,] as practicing clinicians, to integrate and reinforce the application of biostatistical and epidemiologic principles in the evaluation and management of individual patients."[19] The document suggested the following strategy for implementation: have faculty members who both conduct research and teach clinical work write practice books on how to implement epidemiologic methods in medical practice. For example, Sackett and Baskin's (1971) publication of *Methods of Health Care Evaluation* includes materials such as video recordings and written resources pertinent to health care education and evaluation.

The emergence of CE&B and its objectives coincided with that of the medical program. Drafts of "Objectives of the Faculty of Medicine of McMaster University" were primarily spearheaded by Sackett but emerged from collaboration among faculty members who, between 1966 and 1972, engaged in circulating memoranda and sharing drafts of the statement. The primary objective was "to educate," to provide an undergraduate program that could produce students who "are effective solvers of biomedical problems as a result of understanding principles essential to the solution of such problems and knowing how to seek out and use whatever information is required for their solution."[20] The goals of the program were to create students who would "apply fundamental knowledge to clinical problems and participate in the clinical phase of medical education."[21] Last, there was an aim to provide clinicians with the necessary skills for "solving clinical problems through the application of clinical skills and judgment, relating clinical problems to fundamental knowledge, and demonstrating appropriate attitudes toward their own continuing educations and toward the moral and ethical problems facing physicians in relations to patients, colleagues and society."[22] The priorities of continuing medical education programs were understood as a "personal responsibility of clinicians," and it was thought that they would respond to the problem of the gap between medicine and research. The goal of these programs was to "shorten the time between the [scientific discovery] of new knowledge and its safe application to clinical practice."[23]

The research objectives of the program would be in the following areas: biomedical, applied medical research and clinical investigation, and operation research "on health care as [a] guide to educational programmes and [the] use of scarce health personnel."[24] Additionally, the program's strong focus on conducting research to examine "the function of the health team so as to align education programmes with the individual's role" reflected the growing need, as articulated by the relations of discourse, for research relevant to the individual clinician.[25] The "Objectives" document also stated the importance of the collaboration between CE&B and the medical program.[26] The epidemiological research produced by CE&B would not only be relevant to the medical program but would also ensure that the program's rationale would be based on the outcomes of medical research. In other words, the curriculum itself was subject to the same problematizations of practice and outcomes, and the use of scientific methods could verify its effectiveness. In fact, as I discuss later in this chapter, members of the department conducted research on their new approach.

CE&B also created the "Educational Objectives in the Undergraduate Medical Curriculum," which stated that students were to be "concerned with mechanisms of general applicability rather than with content areas related to specific disease."[27] Students would be evaluated based on their proficiency in course objectives and curriculum and by their ability to identify probabilities for understanding the "causation" of disease.[28] Students were also expected to have knowledge of demographic or "situational" factors for predicting disease behaviour.[29] By implementing these goals for medical education, the ideal student would be one who understood medicine on the basis of epidemiologic probabilities (e.g., for diagnosis, or that a treatment would be successful, etc.). The final "Revised Statement of General Goals – MD Program" states that the student is expected "to be able to *critically assess* professional activity related to patient care, health care delivery, and medical research."[30]

The objectives of the medical program and its strategies for implementation were responses to needs for linking clinical practice to its scientific basis in medical research. Between research design and teaching objectives, the McMaster medical program set out on what would become the successful reform of medical training and practice. The primary innovation in curriculum execution was the problem-based method, whereby the training of students targeted their decision-making capacities "to become effective solvers of biomedical problems," and this required that students *learn* how to read and use the literature *at the bedside*.

Concrete Establishments: Conditions for Success

Now that I have explained how problematizations of clinical judgment that concerned the link between laboratory knowledge and bedside practices came to organize the program and resources development at McMaster, I want to discuss the material conditions for the production of knowledge and explain the construction of new social spaces for medical education. Foucault's genealogical work not only aims to spell out the relations of discourse but also to show the "multiplication ... of causes" that explain the production of knowledge in institutional practices: "This procedure of causal multiplication means analyzing an event according to the multiple processes that constitute it" (Foucault 2003, 249). In this subsection I describe the effects and supports of power relations that played a role in organizing emerging training practices at the McMaster medical school.

Throughout the 1970s, health care was a broad political concern. There was significant capital investment from the Ontario Health Resources Development Plan, totalling $640 million [$3 billion]. The objective of this initiative was to increase education research and service requirements and to increase physicians' involvement in training and teaching.[31] The funds would be distributed throughout universities in accordance with the implementation of priorities, such as education. Of this grant, McMaster would receive $103 million [$721 million].[32]

Government documents also contained concerns about scarce resources for training the currently employed professional. At the time, many solutions were offered, and they built on the recommendations made in the report titled *Royal Commission on Health*

Services. To demonstrate the widespread acknowledgment of this problem of training and "scarce resources," in 1964, the same year that *Royal Commission on Health Services* was published, the United States Department of Health, Education and Welfare published *Medical Education Facilities*. This report detailed the importance of site planning and related considerations for the construction of medical training hospitals and facilities. It recommended that the teaching hospital be placed on the same site as the clinical science facilities to make both relevant to medical training. The sites for training medical practitioners would come to be the university hospitals, thus connecting new knowledge with existing forms of training and implementation. The McMaster medical facilities were developed in light of these issues and with support from a large financial investment from the government.

The opening of the McMaster medical school depended on the creation of training facilities. McMaster proposed to build a new health sciences building, the university hospital, where research and clinical training would be intertwined with architectural design. Its first class of incoming students was scheduled for the fall of 1969.[33] The McMaster Health Sciences building would combine primary patient care (four hundred in-patient beds) with an architectural design that joined medical research, a health sciences library, and the clinic. Construction on the building began in 1968 and was completed in 1971, and it cost $56,918,000 [$373 million].[34] (See Figures 1a and 1b.)

The problematization of clinical judgment in health care called for the solutions that McMaster proposed for ameliorating medical training. It was the reconfiguration of the teaching hospital that allowed for the institutional installation of clinical epidemiology, which would later lead to EBM. Medicine would be practised in physical space by combining the hospital, instruction and training, and research spaces: "The building was designed to bring into close proximity the programmes for the various health professions and to integrate the facilities for education and research with those for patient care and clinical investigation."[35] The solution to the "gap" between medical practice ("the clinic") and research ("evidence") was proposed by clinical epidemiology: it was necessary for the two departments to be – concretely – in the same proximity.

The June 1971 issue of *Forum* magazine published a portfolio of the new teaching hospital at McMaster and referred to it as "decentralized education": "The unconventional teaching program at McMaster was a major influence on the design. The medical students will be exposed, from practically the first day of their training, to actual health care functions ... The effect of this program on the building plans is evident. Patient care and research facilities share the same floors."[36]

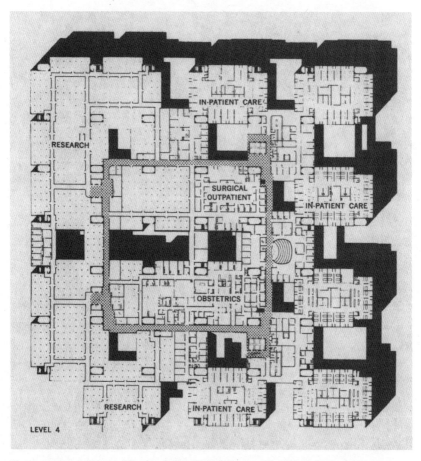

FIGURES 1A AND 1B   Floor plan of McMaster Health Sciences Centre

Source: Archives of Ontario, RG 32-23, box B356178, 1971. June newsletter of *Forum*.

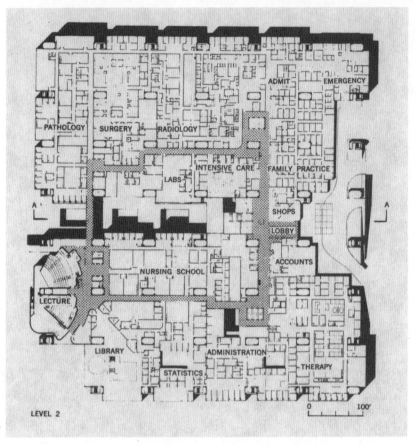

FIGURES 1B   Continued

In an unpublished paper written on the history of the McMaster program, Evans stated that "the Medical Centre represents the physical symbol of many of the principles" articulated in the Faculty of Medicine's "Objectives" statement.[37] The development of a medical centre that placed patient care, education, and research within the same "geographical proximity" was meant to "encourage their integration": "Students from the outset will be oriented to human problems with the focusing of scientific attention on the problems of disease and the translation of research advances into routine clinical service."[38] The space was constructed for flexibility and integration, and it was designed to include the possibility of reorganizing the delivery of care should the needs or foundations for those services change, or should a need arise for restructuring the economy of its operation. There was much debate between the architectural planning and the medical program faculty about the design of the new building. In personal correspondence to Dr. T. McKeown, Evans described the building as "designed to provide close working relationships for clinical and non-clinical departments and to integrate effectively the patient care, educational and research responsibilities of the clinical staff."[39] Sackett echoed the significance of the building's geography in a letter to Mr. E.H. Zeidler: the proximity of CE&B to the other departments was necessary in order for it "to function effectively as a teaching and research unit of the Faculty of Medicine."[40] For Sackett, it was important to ensure the close relationship between the medical staff and, specifically, the department of CE&B so as to maintain the latter's relevance to actual clinical practice. In an early draft of the floorplan design, CE&B was situated separately from the Faculty of Medicine and in-patient care. In a letter to G.P. Hiebert, Sackett complained about the preliminary design plans for the new facility, stating that proximity was a priority: "The crucial relationship for the clinical epidemiologist is his continuing clinical relevancy."[41] The design plans were changed to bring CE&B into the Faculty of Medicine.

The design of the hospital played a major role in the institutionalization of the relations of discourse. In *Discipline and Punish*, Foucault (e.g., 1979, 172–73) spells out, as a means of effective training, the role of architecture in rendering the examination of individuals visible. Building structures are designed to "transform individuals: to act on those it shelters, to provide a hold on their conduct, to carry the effects of power right to them, to make it possible to know them, to alter them" (172). Foucault traces this form of design to the hospital building, whose architecture, over the seventeenth century, had come to allow for greater observation and examination of patients: "The old form of inspection, irregular and rapid, was transformed into a regular observation that placed the patient in a situation of almost perpetual examination" (186).

The architecture of the McMaster Health Sciences complex, also organized around the regular examination of patients, came to include the regular examination of clinical judgments. By placing clinical epidemiology, the science of clinical judgment, right next to the spaces where those judgments happened at the bedside, a new form of observation could be conducted. Students trained in these spaces, and the role of clinical epidemiology in designing the medical school program and curriculum, would also be able to discipline and train new students by perpetually observing their learning in situ.

The new teaching hospital combined, among other things, laboratory research, statistical science, and patient care. The placement of these practices in the same space also provided the conditions for students to learn to make clinical judgments by combining epidemiological and biostatistical knowledge with medical examination. Students' education and training were formed through these practical experiences in the teaching hospital, and so "learning to judge" through the relations of discourse established in clinical epidemiology, and now in social space, could be both effected and supported by this emerging mode of reasoning.

Funding Applied Problems

The decades leading up to the Evidence-Based Medicine Working Group's first statements regarding EBM were heavily influenced by the initial objectives of the Faculty of Medicine, the design and construction of the Health Sciences Centre, and other concrete developments that ensured the continued success of clinical epidemiology. Initiatives that emphasized the *application* of medical science to the bedside were funded by the government and other agencies to support the new focus on applied medical and epidemiological science in clinical care. For instance, in the late 1960s, the Ontario government invested $600 million [$4.5 billion], with an additional $175 million [$1.3 billion] of federal funding, to create regional health centres at the five Ontario medical schools.[42] Following the McMaster research program, these centres conducted local research on the effectiveness of health care services and strategies from a clinical epidemiologic perspective.

An increase in funding support signifies the growing interest in applied research in the health sciences. In 1971, the same year that the Health Sciences Centre opened, Sackett received a National Health Grant to create a health care research centre for training clinical epidemiologists and health care research workers through a series of seminars in health care evaluation methods.[43] The seminars were to be held at McMaster beginning in November of that year. Seminar titles included "The Use of Vital Statistics and Demographic Information in the Measurement of Health and Health Care Needs" and "Randomized Controlled Trials in Health Care."[44] These seminars not only facilitated the clinicians' abilities to fulfill their responsibilities to continue their education post-graduation but also provided instruction on the relevance and uses of clinical epidemiology research in clinical practice.

In 1971, McMaster also received special permission from the Ontario government to create the master of science program in Health Sciences – this at a time when there was an embargo on new programs in Ontario. Despite scarce resources in the Ministry of Education, H.H. Walker, deputy minister of education, wrote that the decision to invest in the new program was due to the "need for qualified people to study diagnostic and therapeutic processes as well as the broad range of basic developmental and highly applied problems related to health."[45] The embargo was originally enforced because of the 1968–69 budget announcement, which affected operating cost grants for universities.[46] There was a lot of support for the new program at McMaster, and its successes can largely be attributed to the significant investments that funding agencies and the provincial government made in its facilities and its programs.

Funding support from international and external sources was another thing that contributed to enabling clinical epidemiology to intervene in clinical care. In the United States, Kerr White assumed the role of deputy director for health sciences at the Rockefeller Foundation. While serving at Rockefeller, White, a critic of "laboratory medicine," gained a reputation for funding studies in clinical epidemiology, a new and emerging field that he saw as promising a better way of practising medicine (Daly 2005, 46). The International Clinical Epidemiology Network (INCLEN) was one such investment. In 1980, INCLEN created a training program whose "goal [was] to strengthen national health care systems and improve health practices globally by providing professionals in the field with the tools to analyze the efficacy, efficiency, and equity of interventions and preventive measures" (INCLEN 2013).

McMaster, specifically the CE&B department, was one of the three leaders in program development and advanced research and training for INCLEN. Thanks to a large financial investment from the Rockefeller Foundation, INCLEN would go on to create clinical epidemiology units (CEUs): "[The] role of the CEU is to promote rational decision-making and the application of quantitative measurement principles ... in the development of clinical and health care policy" in developing nations.[47] CEUs would provide training in the methods of clinical epidemiology so as to facilitate program and policy development in targeted developing regions. The program was funded by the United States Agency for International Development, the World Health Organization, and the International Development Research Centre (in addition to the Rockefeller Foundation).

The first INCLEN meeting was attended by representatives from McMaster, Newcastle University (UK), and the University of Pennsylvania (USA). According to the meeting agenda, the purpose of INCLEN was to bring "Third World" clinical faculty to "developed countries" for training in CEUs, which would produce clinicians who would be "better able to identify and evaluate significant health problems within their own countries."[48] Although INCLEN's focus was global, the program itself sought to improve clinical care at local levels through the use of clinical epidemiology.[49] The funding of this major international project supported the proliferation of the McMaster curriculum. The methods of clinical epidemiology were applied to clinical care worldwide by developing a network of scholars that would resolve population health problems pertaining to the needs of the participant's home country. INCLEN continues to operate, demonstrating the ongoing international significance of clinical epidemiology in medical training and practice.

All the way through the 1980s, members of the department individually conducted successful research programs, holding over $14 million [$35.6 million] in grants from external and internal funding.[50] Other local programs contributed to the success of clinical epidemiology and its stabilization at McMaster and elsewhere. Throughout the 1980s, the CE&B held continuing education classes on the "Critical Appraisal of the Medical Literature." The goals of these classes anticipated the basic premise of EBM, which is that the use of medical literature can productively contribute to the improvement of clinical care. The stated objectives for these continuing education classes called "for the participant to understand and be able to apply to the medical literature some straightforward guides for assessing clinical evidence."[51] The classes facilitated the training of already licensed physicians, introducing them to the new methods of clinical practice at McMaster. New practitioners would be exposed to clinical epidemiology and the critical appraisal method. New and established physicians were the target participants of these new programs, which, through new curricula, sought to intervene in medical education.

Evidence-Based Medicine: McMaster and Beyond

This section explores the links between McMaster, its curriculum, research in EBM, and the various international organizations that influenced and were influenced by McMaster. The medical school curriculum at McMaster was revised in the years prior to the first EBM statements. In the "Department of CE&B Five-Year Overview 1986–1991," the years immediately preceding the first statements of EBM, the department redefined its research objectives. In addition to improving methodological design, measurement, and evaluation in medical research and health services evaluation, the department sought

> to develop new knowledge of the extent to which health care interventions, procedures or services do more good than harm to those, a) who fully comply with recommendations or treatment (efficacy); [and] b) to whom it is offered (effectiveness) ... To develop new knowledge in the application of evidence to specific patient or health problems from the perspective of the health practitioners or policy makers (implementation).[52]

The measures of efficiency and effectiveness are evidence of the prominence of the Cochrane Collaboration and its databases. The education objectives for the CE&B program included developing health professionals who could apply research "to the solution of a broad range of basic, developmental and applied problems related to health care and to use such information to recommend appropriate policies in health and health care."[53] The application of evidence (clinical epidemiologic evidence) to individual patients was justified by recourse to the implementation of policy programs for patient care.

In 1992, the EBM Working Group (EBMWG) at McMaster published its first statements concerning how evidence for clinical judgments should come from scientific study, thus eliminating the contested nature of clinical practice and the fallibility of physician authority or "intuition." The principles of clinical epidemiology that emerged in the 1980s informed the development of EBM. EBM has been said to ask "how methods developed in epidemiology can be effectively applied to bring greater certainty to clinical decision making" (Daly 2005, 24; cf. Fletcher, Fletcher, and Wagner 1982, 82). To paraphrase Feinstein: "The answer to clinical uncertainty lay in science" (Daly 2005, 27). EBM proposed that the methods of the sciences, particularly the systematic assessment of evidence, would provide better and more reliable evidence than individual expertise or intuition.[54] The rules for the systematic assessment of evidence are organized according to the principles of science. EBM argued that the methods for the appraisal of available evidence would become part of the dedicated curriculum of medical practice and that the implementation of EBM could improve the effectiveness of medical judgments more generally. EBM provided metrics that could answer questions about when evidence was sufficient, adequate, and accurate, and how to implement new treatments.

The Evidence-Based Medicine Working Group

The EBMWG was an initiative that emerged in the department of CE&B. It was later described in a department review as an initiative that was undertaken and tested by Gord Grant, Deb Cook and colleagues as part of the Postgraduate Training Program and in the Department of Medicine. It is a multi-institutional collaboration designed to simplify the transfer of rules of evidence to be used by clinicians in decision making and interpretation of clinical scientific literature. Negotiations have been completed to have a series of articles published in *JAMA*, with peer review. This initiative is expected to have a major influence on North American clinical practice, and will further promote the leadership of the Faculty in educational innovation.[55]

In a few years' time, the individual clinician – their decision making and interpretation of the literature – became the site at which evidence-based measures could be implemented. CE&B also noted that there was growing recognition of EBM beyond North America. As mentioned in the previous section, through Ontario regional centres and INCLEN, respectively, clinical epidemiology and its scientific formulation of the clinic had been spreading both locally and worldwide. CE&B rewrote its mission and mandate immediately following the first publications about EBM.

The departmental mission statement now read that CE&B was created in response to the "generally poor quality of clinical research world-wide, to foster rigorous and scientifically valid clinical research methods and their application in the Faculty ... Our over-riding mission can be summarized as: 'a dedication to effect improvements in health by enhancing the quality of clinical research.'"[56] This mission was undertaken through education, research, and service within the faculty of health sciences. The revised academic mission was as follows:

> Our academic mission seeks to advance knowledge in evaluative sciences related to population health and health care through interdisciplinary research, to disseminate knowledge and facilitate the transfer of research information through University and public educational programs, and respond appropriately to calls for methodologic assistance in order to effect improvements in health and to contribute to the communities we serve.[57]

Following these changes, in 1994 the department implemented four new evidence-based initiatives: 1) the creation of a community outreach program for establishing "evidence-based planning and decision making to better inform research questions in the domains of clinical, health and social policy, and health services research"; 2) the development and approval of a new PhD program in Health Research Methodology; 3) the "establishment of the Canadian Cochrane Centre with colleagues across Canada and internationally to provide better access to the best available evidence for interventions in the health field"; and 4) the development of the Ontario Health Care Evaluation Network (OHCEN), a province-wide network for connecting researchers and decision makers (e.g., policy makers).[58]

The vast proliferation of this interest in applying evidence to particular patients through the individual judgments of clinicians started in 1993 with McMaster's first EBM workshop, "How to Teach Evidence-Based Medicine." The name of this annual initiative was later changed to "How to Teach Evidence-Based Clinical Practice." By 1998, eighty-six participants attended the workshop from as far away as Australia, New Zealand, and Japan. Participants took part in an "intense week-long experience exchanging their perspectives and their own teaching techniques while learning more about critical appraisal of clinical evidence."[59] Workshop enrolments were up to ninety-six full registrations by 2000. The traction that EBM gained in a short span of time is evident in the support it received from both financial commitments and workshop participation. The attendance of individual doctors demonstrates the growing perspective that physicians ought to learn the new evidence-based rules of medicine.

Meanwhile in England ... The Oxford Connection

Building on the idea that problematization begins in local institutional contexts and proliferates, becoming an "anonymous phenomenon" (Osborne, Rose, and Savage 2008), I turn to conversations that were ongoing in England, where major reforms were taking place in medical practice and research, and where there was renewed investment in clinical epidemiology and evidence-based recommendations. In 1971, the Rothschild and Dainton reports, collectively titled *A Framework for Government Research and Development,* were published (Civil Service Department 1971). The reports' major areas of concern were the relationships between financial resources and health services and care in the United Kingdom. What emerged from the Rothschild Report was an emphasis on applied research. The report recommended that the Department of Research and Development in the United Kingdom be restructured towards applied research. The guiding principle of "customer-contractor" relationships would reorganize the allocation of funding. For example, the Medical Research Council, which was in charge of administering competitive funding for medical research, would now be "contracted" by the Department of Health, which would determine the focus areas for research. The new interest in "applied" research was the justification for restructuring in medicine. There was an interest in generating information on specific *outcomes* in health services rather than on the knowledge produced by curiosity-driven research.

The shifting focus on epidemiologically measurable improvements in population health came to influence the production of knowledge itself. The Medical Research Council (MRC) expressed its hesitation about the Rothschild Report's recommendations.[60] The council noted the serious effect restructuring would have on university research and the subsequent difficulties of generating the necessary knowledge to enable the departments to pursue their "periphery research."[61] The MRC argued that the outcomes of knowledge production were not a part of the mandate of the research council: it was the government's responsibility to take the results of scientific research and translate them into policy. The restructuring of health research laid the groundwork for what would later be a large government investment in EBM.

The effects of the Rothschild Report were cited in "Paper for the Department Research Strategy Committee" in 1980, which laid out the directions for the Department of Research and Development for the coming decade. The Rothschild Report reallocated 25 percent of the Medical Research Council budget to the health departments (Civil Service Department 1971). The committee also agreed that any research would be "primarily biomedical in nature."[62] Research concerning the link between health and knowledge would now be administered by the Department of Health.

The emphasis on epidemiological research and health services research (both applied fields) continued throughout the 1980s in the United Kingdom. It was during this time that Iain Chalmers set up the Cochrane Collaboration, whose creation paved the way for the proliferation of EBM. Chalmers was inspired by the work of Archibald Cochrane. In 1972, Cochrane published what has become a well-known work in clinical epidemiology: *Effectiveness and Efficiency*. In this book, Cochrane (1972, 22–25) argues that the RCT is the best form of evidence for measuring/testing therapy in a clinical setting and, subsequently, for improving health care. He calls for a "marked increase in knowledge through applied medical research" (78). Despite being against the recommendations of the Dainton Report (79), he sees a need to implement this form of research (81). He foresees, however, that the evidence from effectiveness research will reduce the freedom of clinicians as their decisions would be based on evidence rather than on their individual expertise or subjective perceptions (81–83).

Cochrane's work has been considered a "jibe" at the discipline of medicine. He is very critical about the basis on which clinicians could make judgments: "It is surely a great criticism of our profession that we have not organized a critical summary, by specialty or subspecialty, adapted periodically, of all relevant randomized controlled trials" (Cochrane 1979, 10–11). One of Cochrane's most damning criticisms is pointed at Chalmers's own specialty of obstetric medicine: Cochrane states that this specialty was the least scientific of all. In 1978, Chalmers became director of the National Perinatal Epidemiology Unit at Oxford. At this time, he met Murray Enkin, a Canadian doctor, at the Maternity Centre Association Conference. Enkin would later spend his sabbatical in Oxford with Chalmers (Cassels 2015, 29), where the two decided to create a database of scientific evidence for obstetric medicine: "A few years after [Cochrane's] death, this [jibe] proved to be the rallying point that led to the creation of the Cochrane Collaboration" (as quoted in Cassels 2015, 26).

Chalmers and Enkin, along with Marc Keirse, worked for ten years between 1979 and 1989 mining medical journals and surveying over forty thousand physicians worldwide for publications about obstetrics (Chalmers, Enkin, and Keirse 1989). They then subjected these articles to the method known as the systematic review, which compares various RCT studies for the best evidence in clinical practice. The first iteration of their work was two volumes titled *Effective Care in Pregnancy and Childbirth*. They also published a paperback, a shorter version of *Effective Care,* so that patients could have access to the results of the latest research on the most effective practices (Cassels 2015, 32). The authors saw that their results would become irrelevant as studies continued to be published, so they turned to computer database technology to keep up to date: hence the creation of the Oxford Database of Perinatal Trials (ODPT), which physicians could turn to for answers to clinical questions in obstetrics. The success of the review was due, in part and simultaneously, to their vast distribution and to demand from practitioners. The reviews, which were delivered in disk form, were written in such a way that practitioners could apply their conclusions directly to their practices. These systematic reviews of controlled trials of perinatal care would be updated regularly, in semi-annual disk issues of an electronic journal known as the Oxford Database of Perinatal Trials.

While McMaster was redesigning medical school curricula to improve the judgments of practitioners by offering them training to scrutinize the literature for answers to biomedical questions that emerged in the clinic, the creation of the Oxford database was a pivotal moment for the improvement of medicine at Oxford. The ODPT provided a resource that could reorganize the activities of the clinic: it used scientific evidence, not just convention or expertise, to support the physician's opinion and made it clear that evidence ought to be based on studies of effectiveness. The ODPT was a new infrastructure that made this kind of intervention possible, thus enabling physicians to improve their judgments and keep them in line with emerging measurements.

The ODPT was also a creative event for the proliferation of EBM. The initiative gained attention worldwide and, in 1992, led to the establishment of the Cochrane Centre at Oxford with funds from the Research and Development Programme of the National Health Service (NHS), then headed by Muir Gray. The name was later changed to the UK Cochrane Centre. The funding approval cited the importance of facilitating "the preparation of systematic reviews of randomized controlled trials of health care" (Cochrane Collaboration 2013). The Cochrane Centre received international accolades in major journals such as the *Lancet* and the *British Medical Journal* (*BMJ*). After the success of the Cochrane Centre, Gray saw another opportunity for international recognition: he was given £5 million [$9.4 million] to invest in new research and development initiatives.[63] The funds emerged from a standing committee set up for the House of Lords in the early 1990s. The committee would report to the Department of Research and Development and was funded by the NHS. The success of the Cochrane Centre paved the way for additional resources to support ongoing initiatives for improving health outcomes through medical research.

In 1994, Muir Gray used the £5 million to create the Centre for Evidence-Based Medicine at Oxford University. He recruited Sackett to serve as the first chair and to develop a clinical epidemiology program in the Department of Medicine, Radcliffe Hospital, University of Oxford. On the heels of the Cochrane Collaboration and the publication of the first EBM statements, Sackett built the Centre for Evidence-Based Medicine (CEBM).[64] One of the first projects undertaken by the centre was the 1995 publication of the first issue of *Evidence-Based Medicine,* an academic journal jointly published by *BMJ* and *Annals of Internal Medicine.* The journal's format features rewritten, structured summaries of research articles with commentary and focuses on translating medical research into recommendations for medical practice. It began by reviewing fifty medical journals written in English, and it now reviews one hundred international journals. Within three years of its first publication, the journal would have over seventy thousand subscriptions.

The Cochrane Collaboration and the CEBM were initiatives that both threatened the authority of medicine and responded to threats against that authority. On one hand, EBM provided what Sackett called "a way to stick it to the man" because it provided students with evidence to question their teachers or those who had reputations for being single-minded about disease:

> The Cochrane Collaboration was an extraordinarily powerful threat against authority. Individuals who had reputations based on "this is the way this disorder must be treated" obviously were terribly threatened by what was going to happen with these young upstarts, and kids, and punks, and even lay people challenging them about what they said must occur in terms of health care. (Cassels 2015, 61)

On the other hand, however, EBM could defend the authority of clinical work by showing that it was scientifically effective. Some professionals endorsed EBM, and this created divisions among physicians; however, it was the funding that was instrumental in securing its success.

As an example of the divisions EBM effected within medicine, consider the editorial titled "Evidence-Based Medicine, in Its Place" (1995), which was authored by critics of EBM and appeared in the *Lancet:*

> Cochrane, a fierce individualist ever at war with people who thought they knew best, would hardly welcome the elitism of much evidence-based medicine, and he would certainly scold the founders of Evidence Based Medicine for so far ignoring trials not reported in English and for boiling down the lively broth of published clinical research to a mere 12 mouthfuls per month. Advocates of evidence-based medicine can now afford to lower their profile to ensure that their evolving ideas find a secure place in medical practice. (*Lancet* 1995, 785)

Sackett replied in collaboration with Gray (and others) in the *BMJ* a few months later:

> Good doctors use both individual clinical expertise and the best available external evidence, and neither alone is enough. Without clinical expertise, practice risks becoming tyrannised [*sic*] by evidence, for even excellent external evidence may be inapplicable to or inappropriate for an individual patient. Without current best evidence, practice risks becoming rapidly out of date, to the detriment of patients. (Sackett et al. 1996, 71)

EBM proponents have tried to eliminate elitism by writing articles for *Evidence-Based Medicine* in accessible and nonspecific language. The debate seems, however, to be over the nature of the "problem" of evidence-based medicine: When treating patients, how much should one follow the evidence provided and the recommendations associated with it? The question points to the site of the problem: the individual judgments of practising clinicians.

Since its creation, CEBM has run workshops and courses for training practitioners in the methods of EBM. For example, CEBM holds an annual Evidence Live workshop (it began in 2010) that targets the following medicine-related audiences: academics, clinicians, administrators and managers, private and not-for-profit organizations, and students. The two-day workshops are designed for anyone interested in evidence-based health practice, and they are put on by CEBM. The centre's operating budget, although originally funded by NHS, now depends completely on the tuition fees of participants in courses and workshops. The research carried out at the centre is funded by individual researcher grants rather than by money provided by Oxford.

Institutional Support: Canada and Beyond

Other influences that enabled the proliferation of the EBM program include the immense institutional support found in Canada, the United States, and the United Kingdom. Here I briefly touch on some of the major initiatives, funded by various medical societies, that supported the EBM program and show how these countries contributed to its dominance.

In Canada, the creation of Centres for Health Evidence (CHE) in 1999 was funded by a Canadian National Health Infoway grant in the provinces of Manitoba and Alberta. The CHE's mandate was to "help health practitioners know what to do because quality health information is assembled, integrated and packaged" for direct practitioner use.[65] Further, the Canadian Task Force on Preventive Health Care (CTFPHC), which was created in 1976, officially adopted EBM methodologies in 2002 as well as the grading system for establishing confidence in various evidence-based recommendations.[66] Also in 2002, the Canadian Medical Association began publishing recommendation statements from the CTFPHC online.[67] These major endorsements by various national institutions of medicine in Canada signify the growing dominance of EBM methodologies.

Additionally, Gordon Guyatt created and developed a medical resource called UpToDate. UpToDate was heralded as the first system for evidence-based health care, and it focused on evidence for the management of care, as opposed to previous systems that emphasized evidence relating to physiology.[68] The medical profession's confidence in the solutions to the problems of clinical practice are evident in the use of EBM in medical societies and the subsequent creation of databases that were structured to facilitate the uptake of evidence-based health care recommendations.

These initiatives reach beyond Canada, as already noted. The importance of translating medical research into practice at broader political and institutional levels in Canada was parallelled in the United States and the United Kingdom. The *Journal of the American Medical Association* launched *JAMA Evidence*. The online resource continues to offer textbooks and computerized applications. It is also a searchable database that enables clinicians to "integrate the best evidence with clinical experience" (American Medical Association 2013). The creation of *JAMA Evidence* followed the series of articles that Guyatt published in *JAMA* on how to use the medical literature.

Additionally, in 1999, the United Kingdom created the National Institute for Health and Care Excellence (NICE) to "put guidance into practice" by providing a series of implementation tools, which included the publication of national clinical practice guidelines for various illnesses and procedures. NICE's (2013) focus is on improving health outcomes through evidence-based recommendations in order to "prevent, diagnose and treat disease and ill health." The creation of a government body to reformulate and intervene in medical practice stands as an example of the implementation of EBM in actual practice.

Multiplicity of Causes: The Social Conditions of Success

The emergence of clinical epidemiology was an attempt to merge the scientific foundations of biomedicine and statistics with the clinical judgments made by individual doctors. The creation of new medical databases provided the "evidence" necessary for bringing scientific knowledge into clinical practice. Additionally, the rationale for creating the Faculty of Medicine at McMaster relied heavily on the relevance of epidemiological methods for clinical practice. The Health Sciences Centre at McMaster institutionalized the solutions proposed by clinical epidemiology: it placed research and training side by side in a social space, and it facilitated the revision of medical training more generally. These conditions allowed clinical epidemiology and, later, EBM to become the predominant method for medical education and practice.

Seeing the broader contingent connections between the discursive concerns and the material conditions that allowed the McMaster curriculum to stabilize and proliferate sheds light on the relations of power that structure the relationships between different actors in health care: physicians, medical students, researchers, government, and other providers. The problems associated with clinical judgment were generative of new methods of thought for proposing new lines of action. It depended on political, economic, and social relations to stabilize in the institution. Without an emerging database of evidence, there may not have been the resources for clinicians to learn to use evidence. Without a space that combined new methods of reasoning with patient care, students may have never learned to integrate these two domains of practice. These conditions resulted in the constitution of specific forms of subjectivity, which I discuss in the next chapter.

3

Responsibilizing a New Kind of Clinician: Problem-Based Learning

In this chapter I show that the medical program at McMaster used the problem-based learning (PBL) teaching model to create a new kind of student. PBL connected the facts from medical science with clinical work by training students to ask a clinical question and then look to the literature to resolve it. Research from clinical epidemiology concerning clinical effectiveness served to found and justify this new curriculum. Classified as a new skill set, PBL was about "the acquisition of an integrated knowledge base" (Barrows 1996, 6). PBL pioneered a new way of training clinicians: "When it was introduced there was no philosophical or cognitive theoretical underpinning explicitly stated by the founders of the McMaster Medical School" (Neville 2009, 1). It was a method used to combine information from clinical epidemiology with practice.

While the previous chapter explains how the McMaster Health Sciences Centre institutionalized the solutions to the problematization of clinical judgments in the reorganization of material space, this chapter shifts its genealogical focus to explain how the institutionalized practices associated with educational training effected subjectivity: Who was the target of these new strategies of training and how were they conceived? Because the architecture of the new teaching hospital allowed for the observation and examination of clinical judgment via the programmatic science of clinical epidemiology, the strategies and relations of discourse constituted a specific kind of subject within the medical training program. I argue that these new modes of training had consequences for physician responsibility. McMaster sought to move beyond a traditional division of labour in the teaching hospital and conceived of a new student who learned not only the conventional aspects of biomedical knowledge but also what other professions did, which constituted a genuine focus on inter-professional training. Because the emphasis was on the fact that information was different and always changing, the responsibility of the physician to make the best judgment based on the best available evidence became tantamount. The student had to become a lifelong learner, and this responsibility to keep up was installed in various aspects of the training program.

To present EBM as part of a concrete social apparatus, I analyze the relations of discourse and the strategies that came to organize particular forms of conduct. In order to understand the effects of these intersecting relations on the constitution of the subject, I conceptualize the object of medical training as the thing on which power relations work to ameliorate clinical judgment. Within the relations of discourse, the student's subjectivity and her/his knowledge and conduct in the clinic become the target of the new program at McMaster. To spell out the elements of the dispositif, I articulate the forms of subjectivity that are constituted by the relations of discourse and the strategies of conduct (cf. Deleuze 1992, 159). To conceptualize the subject, I follow Foucault's (2000, 327) method: "We have to know the historical conditions that motivate our conceptualization." In order to understand the concept of the lifelong learner, a key objective of the McMaster program, I provide an account of the historical conditions that brought this idea to life. In the end, the McMaster program subjected students through a form of self-knowledge (cf. Deleuze 1999, 103). I draw on the work of Alan Hunt to explain how this form of self-knowledge – that is, the creation of the lifelong learner – constituted a form of responsibilized subjectivity. I show not only how these techniques individualized students to become self-learners and to keep up with the knowledge within the clinical sciences beyond graduation but also how this linked up with new initiatives at the levels of national education and provincial regulation.

Problem-Based Learning: Training a New Kind of Clinician

Before exploring the implementation of PBL in the McMaster medical program, I must explain what it is. Harold S. Barrows was a member of the McMaster medical school faculty and, over his career, he wrote extensively about its new curriculum. In one of his published articles about the teaching methods created by the instructors at McMaster, Barrows (1996, 3) states that McMaster had implemented new techniques of medical training that would come to influence other schools worldwide. What has come to be known as the problem-based learning method is said to have its roots in educational psychology, which focuses on the study of development and knowledge.

In a 1979 report prepared for and distributed by the National Institutes of Health, Barrows and Tamblyn (the latter a clinical lecturer in nursing at McMaster) define PBL as "the individualized learning that results from working toward the *solution* or *resolution* of a problem" (emphasis in original). In their model, the problem is the stimulus for learning or collecting facts about a problem. Problems are typically clinical in nature insofar as they deal with actual patient concerns, which allows for the development of "clinical (or diagnostic) reasoning (also referred to by such terms as: medical inquiry skills, problem-solving skills, and clinical judgment)." The immediate educational goal is to stimulate student learning and acquire the skills necessary to collect *useful* information about the problems that patients present with. They see clinical reasoning as the most important skill physicians have, and they define it as the "many skills necessary to evaluate and manage patient problems effectively, efficiently, and humanely" (Barrows and Tamblyn 1979, 1). Here the notion of critical evaluation or appraisal of information can be observed, as can Cochrane's exact language on effectiveness and efficiency. The PBL method is a solution to the problems of health outcomes problematized in the literature and discussed in the preceding chapter.

PBL, the authors of the report argue, is the best method for synthesizing information from a variety of health disciplines and enabling students to learn and apply it appropriately. Their model was a reaction to the "pattern technique," whereby, "similar to a computer, a clinician stores complete constellations of symptoms and signs in his [*sic*] head to be cued, by association, to the patient's complaints and findings" (Barrows and Tamblyn 1979, 9). Instead, they suggest that the astute physician learns how to keep her mind open to various possibilities, to distill the problem by ruling in and ruling out which details are relevant to her diagnosis, and to come to various hypotheses about what is causing the patient's complaints. PBL, they reason, reduces potential medical harms because it effectively finds the causes.

There are different models of PBL. I offer a general description of these variations and then show how the McMaster curriculum deployed PBL to reform medical education so as to resolve the problematized aspects of clinical practice. The first step to designing the PBL method is to "decide on desired educational objectives and then select the method that fits best" (Barrows 1986, 485). The McMaster program sought to train students to solve biomedical problems, which required the development of "clinical reasoning skills" – that is, solving clinical problems with critical thinking (Barrows 1983, 3078). Barrows argues that "this method facilitates the integration of knowledge from the separate disciplines into an organized knowledge base useful in solving clinical problems" (ibid.). McMaster's curriculum made clinical epidemiology a fundamental component in its training and learning environments. The use of the PBL method allowed students to learn to combine information from clinical epidemiology and biostatistics – research that measured the effectiveness of clinical intervention – and to apply it directly in their decision-making and reasoning processes.

PBL comprises the assembly of a variety of components and steps. Medical school students are assigned to tutorial groups.

Each meeting begins with a problem, such as a case history or clinical vignette (Barrows 1986). This method is carried out during the preclinical years so that students learn to integrate textbook knowledge into their decision making. During the tutorial, students try to figure out the mechanisms that cause the symptom(s) presented in the problem vignette. The assumption underpinning this method is that student "understanding precedes rational action, both in education and in practice" (Schmidt 1983, 13). If students understand the scientific facts about the biomedical mechanisms, they are able to make judgments about what might be causing the presenting symptoms. After they try to figure out the nature of the problem and a hypothesis for its cause, they begin an inquiry (such as by looking at lab tests, conducting an examination). Once they receive new information, they return to their groups to review their hypotheses, converse, and challenge each other's assumptions. Once the group reaches a consensus, students record what they need to review from their lecture notes, textbooks, and so on, "areas in which learning is needed to develop better hypotheses, to improve approaches for analyzing data and synthesizing the problem, and to make better decisions as to the underlying mechanisms responsible for the patient's problem" (Barrows 1983, 3079). PBL emphasizes self-directed evaluation, encourages students to become self-directed learners both during the tutorial and after, and affects how they make decisions and how they tackle the presented problem along the way (a method Barrows [1986, 484] refers to as closed-loop PBL).

Others have described PBL in more "meta" terms. Schmidt's (1983, 13–15) procedure requires that tutorial groups first clarify the concepts they need to understand in order to assess the problem. Next, students need to know which phenomenon needs to be explained. In the clinic students will have to know how to formulate a question for which they will need to seek information, according to the McMaster curriculum. After they formulate relevant hypotheses, students would then evaluate whether the possible causes of the process with which they are concerned are correct and complete. The members of the group would then formulate learning objectives (i.e., they would determine what it is they are seeking information about). For example, if, in a vignette, a patient is coughing blood, the group needs to determine the difference between a cough reflex and, say, lung cancer. Students divvy up tasks for individual study, and when they return to the group, they synthesize knowledge, test new information, and together review the steps in their reasoning.

PBL was a solution to the problem of the application of knowledge in the clinic. The education curriculum was designed on the basic understanding that "people can possess knowledge which they seem unable to apply" (Schmidt 1983, 11). Barrows's original article published in *JAMA* draws on the problematization of education to justify McMaster's new curriculum of medical education. This form of self-directed learning aims "to increase the retention of facts and their recall in the clinical situation" (Barrows 1983, 3077). In the original article in which he coined the term "PBL," Barrows posed the problem with current training methods as one related to the rapidly changing world of medicine: "Much of what they [instructors] do teach will be forgotten, become out of date, or be incorrect in the future. Independent, self-directed learning is another skill that must be learned in medical school, since there will be no lectures, syllabi, or reading assignments after graduation" (ibid.). Barrows also noted that a number of medical associations were pointing a spotlight at medical school curricula and highlighting old methods that are no longer effective or efficient for the present-day medical system. For example, both the Macy Conference on the Teaching of the New Biology and the Conference on Future Directions of Health Professions Education recommended that there "should be more emphasis on independent study and problem solving" (ibid.). Becoming independent learners meant that students would be lifelong learners, committed to enhancing their knowledge and continuing their medical education well beyond graduation: "In this process, the students are provided the skills necessary to recognize their learning needs and to expand or modify the knowledge they acquire in the future, as appropriate, through self-directed learning" (3078). At McMaster, students were to take "responsibility for their own education."[1] Independent learning would continue to be a concern through the 1980s (e.g., see Barrows 1996, 4) and also in the early days of the McMaster curriculum.

In this chapter, I first explicate the notion of the individual clinician as lifelong learner. I provide the background for the creation of the McMaster program and how PBL organized its pedagogy and teaching methods. After describing the four phases of the program and the new "clerkship" (which would come before the residency), I show how the program's focus also shifted to the idea of training the physician's "attitude." This focus on what was termed a "horizontal program" in medical education recasts the student's responsibility to their own learning. I also explain how students were disciplined and evaluated in order to facilitate the development of a personal duty to self-learning through an engagement with the literature on responsibilization.

The Subject of Medical Education

The success of the PBL method relied on the emerging concept of the physician that figured in the new field of clinical epidemiology. Doctors needed to be trained to use scientific knowledge in their practices in order to improve the effectiveness of bedside care. The McMaster medical school sought to instill this duty in their trainees, to get them to understand that their jobs were not only informed by science but also required them to keep up with that science. This meant two things: 1) doctors at McMaster were conceived of as solvers of biomedical problems; and 2) doctors would have to learn how to keep up with the medical literature so that their knowledge would never go out of date. In order to avoid conventionalism, which was thought to plague the problems associated with poor medical practice, doctors would have to see it as their personal responsibility to update their knowledge and improve their practice throughout their careers. In other words, they would have to become "lifelong learners." In order to understand how the PBL method was designed to idealize physicians as problem-solvers – something that first served to remedy the disjuncture between the increasingly fast advances in the laboratory and the lag time between that and clinical practice, and later served to show that making the best judgments required keeping up with the advances of medicine and best evidence – I first discuss the medical program at McMaster. In doing this I expose how the tactics of education were deployed not only to improve medical judgments but also to render the new doctor responsible for making better judgments.

Background: A New Method for Self-Learning

The McMaster medical program had four phases and a clerkship prior to residency training (which, in Canada, was regulated by the provincial colleges). It also had what was termed a "horizontal program." This was "new" in that it aimed to respond to a number of growing concerns in the field of medical education. In a planning document, the program development committee justified the need to abandon conventional training methods:

> Current dissatisfaction with medical education imposes on a new medical school a responsibility to experiment with novel approaches ... The planners of the M.D. curriculum in Canada's fourteenth medical school have responded to the urge to innovate and the reader can appreciate the spirit of our planning if he [*sic*] accepts modification or change as the only constant.[2]

Direct reference is made to the identified need to reform medical education in a time of rapidly changing information.

The pedagogy of the program was organized around the following principle: disease was more than just discomfort or disability – it was a "deviation from health."[3] This meant that a fundamental knowledge in biology would be required by students insofar as they needed to understand how to use concepts and to develop an "approach for research and practice concerning prevention, diagnosis and rehabilitation."[4] The program's priority was to train students in the science of human biology while simultaneously getting them to see how that knowledge was critical for bedside practice: "As students become accustomed to the approach and realize what is expected of them, they will choose their own approaches to problems and become increasingly adept at planning, informing themselves and reporting conclusions."[5] From early on, the program planners sought to encourage students to develop their capacities for clinical judgment based on the link between science and care, and to "inform themselves" rather than simply being passive in their learning.

The program was conceived with two objectives in mind. The first objective was quite concrete: "To help students become effective solvers of biomedical problems by understanding the principles essential to the solution of such problems, and by learning how to seek out and use what information is required."[6] Not only must students learn how to apply information, but they must also learn how to know what information they should seek out. The second objective concerns something a bit abstract: "To foster attitudes to behavior as responsible physicians and scientists in their relation to patients, colleagues, and society."[7] This objective would come to be the topic of much discussion over the early years of the program. The attitude characteristics listed in the planning documents are: compassion, to promote health to the public, and to act ethically in the public good.[8] The difficulties would concern the evaluation of these faculties. These qualities, however, were the focus of the horizontal program (which I discuss later).

The curriculum aimed to fulfill its objectives by means of the PBL method, which would introduce students to clinical problems early on in their training. This method differed from the conventional model of memorizing biological facts, testing knowledge, and then enrolling in residency training. Curriculum planners saw it as of the utmost importance that students see the relevance of learned information to its application in the clinical setting *right from the start*. They saw this as the best way for PBL to foster student motivation and self-understanding: students, they hoped, would learn a "responsible professional attitude."[9] Presenting students

with clinical problems and the impetus to collect and learn biological facts ensured that the relevance of science was clear from the
beginning. The learning environment was also structured along
these lines: "Learning will take place in the context of a series of
major biomedical problems and questions requiring understanding of principles and collection of data by students for their solution."[10] Faculty, then, were not lecturers, they were tutors, guides
to learning what questions to ask and what information to gather.
Students would learn in small groups, be given lab time, and have
access to and be encouraged to use multiple learning resources
(many courses had a computer/technology component).[11] The
method of instruction is described as follows and is in line with
the PBL method:

> The students will be presented with a series of major biomedical
> problems and questions requiring the understanding of princi-
> ples and the collection of data by students approaching their
> solution. In each problem area, the student should be able to
> choose from among a variety of specific problems. This flexibil-
> ity will provide an opportunity for each streaming according to
> individual interests and goals.[12]

Becoming a solver of biomedical problems meant that a student
had to learn how to find relevant information, a skill that program
planners hoped would endure throughout the graduate's career.

During the planning phase of the construction of the Health Sciences Centre at McMaster there were special requests for tutorial
rooms rather than for the conventional lecture halls: "These rooms
should seat six comfortably and in some cases, [and] be equipped
with video-tape viewing equipment."[13] The medical school asked
for thirteen rooms total and also requested the construction of
a film room so students could view audiovisual materials. There
were also learning labs and carrels so that students could have
access to the library's learning resources twenty-four hours a day,
seven days a week. The design of the tutorial rooms and private
learning spaces was meant to organize the learning practices of

students: students would work in small groups, as they would on the wards after graduation, and they would learn to work alone with resource materials so they could develop self-learning skills. As discussed in Chapter 2, these spaces also allowed faculty and tutors to observe and examine the students' judgments in situ. The construction of these spaces provided an architecture to surveille and correct the skills students were practising. These skills required that students knew how to work independently to solve problems and to update their knowledge.

These physical spaces were consistent with the centrality of PBL and its emphasis on the student's responsibility for their own learning. PBL focuses on "the development of self-study skills"; it is the student's responsibility to determine "what is to be learned and how it is to be learned" (Barrows and Tamblyn 1979, 2). In their first publication about the practice and teaching of PBL, Barrows and Tamblyn suggest a checklist that would enable students to ask themselves what information they have or are lacking. One of these questions is: "Do I have sufficient background knowledge to continue working with this problem?" (14). Students were to learn *both* how to self-assess the degree to which their knowledge is sufficient or lacking and how to direct their learning to better their understanding. They were also to know where to find and retrieve information to help them accomplish this objective. Among the resources Barrows and Tamblyn list to help students to learn how to better deal with problems are scholarly sources, laboratory work, and other professionals. The tutor system was another resource for students – one that could teach them how to recognize their skill sets, their knowledge, and their limitations. These, of course, would be improved when students encountered clinical problems of their own.

These types of self-corrective measures can be understood as disciplinary tactics. Foucault's concept of disciplinary power views the body as a machine of made up of forces, and it seeks to optimize these capacities through the tactical use of "simple instruments," including hierarchical observation. According to Foucault's (1979, 170) research, training programs rely on this form of power, and hierarchical observation is "a mechanism that coerces by means of observation." This apparatus makes it possible for the examiner to see the techniques of the program being executed and to evaluate those in training. PBL was exercised by tutors and faculty who could readily observe the capacity of students to assess their knowledge, to make judgments about this knowledge, and to apply it to the problem case. They could also observe which resources the students reviewed, how they interacted with their peers, which faculty members they sought out for advice, and the final assignment they turned in for grading. The training of lifelong learners required that students be constantly supervised by a variety of professionals.

The last principle that organized the PBL curriculum design was the idea that there should be a division of labour among health sciences faculty and that different knowledge users could help solve biomedical problems: "The delivery of health care is a team responsibility shared with many personnel with different types of training," and this presents a "unique opportunity" to train and to learn to work together effectively.[14] The physical space of the health sciences centre was meant to integrate various forms of biomedical knowledge: "The building [health sciences centre] has been designed to bring into close proximity the programs for the various health professions and to integrate the facilities for education and research with those for patient care and clinical investigation."[15] Students would learn to work alongside other practitioners (learning others' roles and responsibilities in addition to their own) and would learn how to seek out relevant information from other providers in order to improve bedside care. The PBL method organized learning around problem-solving, so any clinical "problem" that was presented to students could require them to learn from a number of different health care workers. This aspect of the program was essential for understanding the creation of the clerkship and the elective elements of the program. The more information students could learn about health care delivery, and how different medical evidence could be used to execute care, the more medical judgments would come to be based on the best possible knowledge.

In addition to being involved in hierarchical observation, discipline functions within curricula such as PBL through its fundamental self-corrective measures (cf. Foucault 1979, 179). Discipline pressures its subjects to perform corrective measures when their performance goals have not yet been obtained. PBL requires students to continue to work and to study the materials needed to resolve their case problem until a tutor or faculty member deems it has been addressed in a satisfactory manner. Once the student does this, she or he can go on to other problems and so advance within the program. Discipline, as a force relation, rarely relies on punishment when a skill is performed incorrectly; instead, it coerces through reward. The McMaster program ensures that students are rewarded for seeking out members of health care teams for their advice and expertise. As students are rewarded for their correct conduct within the program, they are able to advance through the program and to practise and perform the skills necessary to self-evaluate and correct their capacities by themselves. In other words, they become self-learners, which is the ultimate goal of the program.

There were many innovative aspects to the design of the program, including the emphasis placed on the students' self-motivation to learn. There was also minimal lecture content, use of multimedia materials to gain access to resources, and a tutor system. I discuss these components in relation to each of the phases. The original program contained four "phases." In Phase I students learned about human biology (e.g., anatomy, genetics, physical examination, normal human behaviour) as well as how to use the resources on campus.[16] These medical students would find themselves on the wards from the earliest days in the program. When the original goals of Phase I were conceived, they included an introduction to the hospital facilities, staff, and laboratories (including learning about the technical skills carried out in the labs).[17] Phase I was also to set the ground work for the principle objective of PBL: "[To] lay the foundation for *self learning* ... [and] Provide a *transitional period* of weaning away from traditional didactic teaching to self learning based on problem solving."[18] Students would also learn how to use the library as a resource for finding information on clinical problems – a skill that could join medical research to application at the bedside as a lifelong activity. The content of Phase I included scientific lab work: learning what goes on in the laboratory meant that students could become familiar with the biological processes of the human body. The overall challenge was to "present the basic sciences in such a way that the boundaries between the laboratory and the clinic are so blurred that the student will learn to depend on this basic knowledge as essential in his [*sic*] practice of medicine."[19] Phase I was about the presentation of clinical materials through clinical teachers, keeping students' motivation to learn high by encouraging them to see diagnosis and physical examination as a result of medical and biological sciences.[20]

Later iterations of the goals of Phase I synthesized problem-solving and self-learning. The most important skill involved in learning to be a physician is learning how to find information to solve clinical problems using medically relevant resources: Phase I "provide[d] an orientation to the technique of self learning based on problem solving and making effective use of tutors, resource persons, library and audiovisual aids."[21] One of the primary methods of instruction was developmental discussion, which resembled PBL insofar as it involved small groups, tutorial leaders, and student-generated information about problems. There were also assigned projects that, for example, asked students to learn "all you can about the thyroid gland."[22] This encouraged students to learn how to gather information on receiving an open-ended question. One of the module's instruction methods dealt with epidemiological materials.[23] Exposing students to knowledge about "risk factors" in different systems of the body was intended to show them how disease outcomes were related and continuous "rather than discrete variables."[24] Group work also allowed students to choose among different sets of problems in the hope that they would be motivated to self-study in accordance with their individual learning goals and interests. Phase I also introduced students to the tutor system, which was their primary method of learning. Tutors led students through the program, and faculty members were seen as guides for each learning unit, while, ideally, students would teach themselves how to learn from medical sciences.[25] Clinical skills, such as learning how to gather information during the clinical encounter, were also taught by faculty in a more traditional, apprenticeship fashion.

During the first review of the medical program in 1972, three "major problems" were highlighted for Phase I. Faculty disagreed among themselves about the objectives of this phase of the program, which had to do with "the difficulties of achieving a content oriented objective in an educational system which is content to emphasize process."[26] Evaluation was also a challenge for tutors and faculty: How could one really assess whether students were meeting their personal learning goals? The PBL method required that they set their own focus and use of time.[27] There were also difficulties with the anatomy section of the program. Dr. George Sweeney wrote about this issue in the review:

> The position of anatomy as a departmental contribution is again somewhat unique because Phase I takes place in the multi-media laboratory within the Department of Anatomy. Problems of two types arise from this situation. First, there are administrative problems in running a properly integrated inter-departmental programme in an area with defined departmental jurisdiction, second, Phase I students and some members of the Anatomy Department do not accept that instruction in anatomy will be adequate if the "self-learning through problem-solving" approach is followed rigidly ... Personally, I do not yet think we have developed problem based learning and its subsequent evaluation to a point where more traditional ways of presenting anatomical data can be abandoned entirely.[28]

There was disagreement about the role of PBL: Should it replace traditional ways of presenting materials? As a result, the general sense of the first review is best summed up as follows: "Phase I is not satisfying many members of this faculty in providing sound education in disciplines such as anatomy and biochemistry regarded as fundamental to medicine."[29] While faculty saw that the objectives were clear and important, there was a lot of trouble with regard to their implementation. These concerns point to the tension between facts and their application even at the level of education reform. Just as the problematization of medical facts as they pertained to the bedside was found in the literature, so, too, did it figure among program design and implementation: What was the role of content in the curriculum? Students and faculty were troubled by this disconnect between what to teach and how to teach it.

While Phase I comprised fourteen weeks of the program, Phase II comprised six weeks of learning about the mechanisms of disease and the function of cells.[30] This phase was almost entirely scientific in nature, and its objective was for students to gain an "understanding of the ways in which the bodily dynamic equilibrium may respond to environmental alterations" as well as to the improvement of self-learning techniques.[31] This phase also incorporated PBL and the tutor system. The first review reported problems with the tutor system: "Some tutors have found difficulty in adjusting to the delicate McMaster tutorial system," which McMaster program planners tried to remedy with 1) a paired tutor system, whereby a novice tutor would be paired with an experienced tutor, and 2) "a special tutor-training program."[32] Faculty found the first solution to be "generally unacceptable" given its demands on their time, while the other approach was "being continued and extended, but there remain[ed] some problem in that tutors most in need of such training [were] sometimes the least enthusiastic attenders."[33] There were many challenges in training tutors to fulfill their role and function in the program. Major areas of concern pointed out by the review had to do with the relevance of medical sciences to medical practice: "Many students continue to have some difficulty, and some students have much, in perceiving the relevance of 'academic' basic science to clinical practice and problems ... It is thought that the solution may lie in greater earlier exposure of the students to live patients as problems."[34] The solution was to involve students in clinical work as soon as possible.

Phase III was a lengthy forty-week curriculum, and it focused on the organ systems, the point at which students would start to integrate their knowledge from the previous units on biology.[35] Its learning goals included the ability for the student to "discern and to approach specialized biomedical problems," "derive on his [*sic*] own and to use most effectively the information he required to approach the solution of these problems," and to understand the various mechanisms that maintain and alter health function of the body.[36] Learning materials in Phase III would be presented in a matrix: students would learn "everything of important clinical relevance" to a system.[37] Here is an example of the learning matrix: "16 students studying diseases of the liver will be divided into groups of four, each with one tutor, not necessarily an expert in this field. It may be an Anatomist whose understanding of the clinical aspects is not deep. This will encourage students to utilize other areas of learning."[38] Learning from "non-experts" was one way that the McMaster program sought to encourage interdisciplinary knowledge sharing.

The objective of Phase III was to position the student to be ready to undertake a clinical clerkship. This format was new to medical education and aimed to execute the principle of integrated professions and knowledge. In a matrix module, students would be exposed to problems with a presenting patient, at which point they would discuss the anatomy of the liver, its systems and functions, using models, scientific slides, pictures, imaging, and so on. Then they would learned how to examine a liver in a presenting patient. Following this, under the guidance of the tutor, students would search the literature for causes of presenting symptoms and do work in multidiscipline labs.[39] The curriculum was designed to bring the student into contact with knowledge from a variety of sciences and professions, and to learn how to apply that knowledge to clinical work. The bridge between the lab and the clinic was to intertwine those activities through physical space and the discursive practices related to seeing patients, saying what system was the cause of the problem, and then finding a solution from the medical and clinical sciences. In the first program review of Phase III, the identified problems had to do with, again, getting students to see the relevance of the link between the sciences and clinical practice: "Several arrangements have been tried to help students use the disciplines and concepts of basic science to enhance their ability to solve problems."[40] The remedy would be sought through greater involvement of "basic science faculty in the planning of problems on which students are to work. [P]roblems can be constructed in a way to lead students into looking into appropriate basic science areas in which these areas are shown to be relevant in a broad context for medicine."[41] There were many issues with implementing the PBL method, but the main concerns were to use it to get students to learn how to see the connection between medicine and science through emphasizing their own responsibility to learn and apply it.

The development of clinical clerkship was a new aspect of the McMaster school and it was premised on the following: if the program was about teaching students to become problem solvers, they would need an opportunity to develop clinical skills before Phase IV and to see that the "link between 'clinical work' and 'basic science' must be constant, direct and meaningful."[42] Phase IV's goals were the following: "To have the clinical clerk act as a functioning member of the health team with responsibility under supervision for a carefully controlled number of patients"; "to enable the student to solve clinical problems by relating them back to basic concepts and knowledge acquired in earlier phases of the curriculum"; to learn about the emotional assets and limitations; to examine skills and "critically evaluate" the findings from this; and, relatedly, to "critically evaluate" the data from lab and imaging tests.[43] This last stage of the program was the ultimate synthesis of knowledge and practice, which occurred while gaining real-world and hands-on experience prior to the residency requirement of the provincial colleges.

Additionally, and consistent with the program focus on critical appraisal, students were also supposed to learn to demonstrate "the ability to critically evaluate the data acquired" in the examination process.[44] The clerkship was eleven months long and, for the first time, students would take responsibility for patient care. The goals of the clerkship included interprofessional teamwork and understanding: "Learn to relate to and communicate effectively with other members of the health team."[45] There was also an emphasis on clinical problems that could be solved by use of biological or scientific information: Students would "encounter clinical problems that call on them to relate back to the concepts and knowledge acquired in the earlier phases, thus emphasizing the importance of fundamental human biology with respect to the problems of patients."[46] The clerkship experience also attempted to deal with emotional dilemmas for both patients and physician. Because students would be seeing live patients, the clerkship allowed them to practise doing the clinical exam and critically appraising the information gathered during this encounter: Students would "develope [*sic*] competence in clinical examination, including history taking, physical examination and a rational understanding of planning, investigation and therapy. As well, [the student] should acquire the ability to critically evaluate the data derived by these processes."[47] Throughout their clerkship, students had compulsory rounds in family practice and other team medicine contexts (including, for example, surgery). Students were also able to use resources like videotape and one-way glass observation to gain more experience with the clinical encounter.

The program review report cited issues with students entering the clerkship feeling inadequately prepared for clinical work.[48] Further, the report stated that there were issues with the integration of departments in the program but that there were ongoing training efforts to help improve communication between the various aspects of the multidisciplinary approach to teaching students.[49] Work was also being done to improve the tutor system, including clarifying the "role of tutors in relation to clinical teachers and evaluators," which would be accomplished through better training, and a workshop was scheduled to facilitate this.[50]

I now discuss another new aspect of the McMaster curriculum, the "horizontal program," before further exploring the tutor system. This further elucidates the personal duty of physicians to become better doctors and to accept that lifelong learning is their responsibility.

The Horizontal Program

Sackett chaired the horizontal program, and it was a unique aspect of the McMaster program. It ran throughout the other phases of the students' medical education and was "devoted to consideration of problems relating to professional attitudes and ethics, abnormal behavior, rehabilitation medicine and the use of biomedical statistics."[51] This subsection explores the integration of medical ethics and professional duties with the medical education program and also spells out the implications for the subject of the McMaster curriculum.

The objectives of the horizontal program were "to foster attitudes and skills leading to [students'] behavior as responsible physicians and scientists in their relation to patients, colleagues, and society."[52] The "vertical program" refers to the academic aspects of medical practice, whereas the "horizontal program" refers to the fact that this program ran for three hours a week throughout the three phases of the curriculum and engaged with questions of "attitudes, feelings, and human values."[53] The primary focus on attitudes refers specifically to "the development of mental dispositions to behave in a certain fashion."[54] The main objectives concerned the ability of students to develop an interest in their patients as "people," to develop long-term relationships with them, and to develop good interviewing skills for clinical examination. Of the six goals of this program, I focus on the following: "To develop a physician who views his responsibility to his patient as a long-term commitment";[55] to develop a sense of professional and social responsibility as a physician; and to "develop a physician who knows himself,"[56] which means a physician who knows her limitations and continues to be a self-learner throughout her career.

As their first responsibility is to the patient, students in the McMaster program needed to develop a sense of compassion and personal commitment to their practice. In 1969, the interim report of the horizontal program included information about its initial planning of curriculum material. A compassion for the health of the patient was understood as a societal goal: "To foster attitudes leading to behavior as responsible physicians and scientists in their relation to patients, colleagues and society. Such behaviour is marked by compassionate concern for patients coupled with action to promote the public good when the physician is faced with ethical decisions."[57] One of the curriculum activities that sought to cultivate this attitude occurred during the clinical clerkship when students were placed on the wards in a number of personally and ethically challenging situations. For example, students would be placed on wards with infants with congenital defects. They would be teamed up with a "preceptor," who would act as a role model regarding how to act in these clinical situations.[58] Being in these situations enabled students to learn about the key ethical dilemmas they would encounter in their interactions with a variety of "abnormal" patients.[59]

When it came to linking the duties of medical practice to social and professional responsibility, the horizontal program tried to give students an understanding of various health relationships, such as the doctor-patient relationship, relationships with other health professionals, relationships with society, and long-term patient relationships as well as the notion of the patient as a "whole person." This meant going beyond physiological health to take into consideration patients' families, environments, jobs, and so on.[60] These responsibilities could be learned through the critical incident approach,[61] which was an aspect of the PBL method whereby students considered the "ethical and value problems" of medical practice by critically reviewing case files.

Further, interprofessional contact was also integrated with medical practice to foster a sense of social and professional responsibility: "The student should demonstrate a knowledge of the precise services provided by these other health professions."[62] Students were also expected to learn how to "participate with other health professionals in the management of the patient as a co-equal, deciding *as a group* who should direct a given phase of this management."[63] Physicians would learn from other faculty how to provide patients with information about other governmental and lay groups relevant to their care. During clinical hours, students were expected to "exhibit behavior in dealing with the patient and his family, other health professionals, health groups, and the general public which is consistent with societally-determined codes of professional and personal conduct."[64] In dealing with matters of professional and social responsibility, the student ought to learn how to appropriately disseminate medical knowledge and to "demonstrate, in his commitments, a respect for alternative points of view, both from his colleagues and from individuals outside the health professions."[65] The main methods of instruction for these forms of clinical attitudes involved pairing students with teachers who would act as "role models." This was because the program planners felt that the appropriate attitudes couldn't be taught merely as "content" or "facts."[66] Two courses, "Medical Practice" and "Issues in Medicine," provided primarily informal settings in which faculty and students could discuss the critical incidents that arose from examining case files or from matters that presented to students during clinical rounds.[67] This model of instruction encouraged students to see their responsibilities with regard to decision making as being part of learning team work. One of the major problems noted in the first report of the Horizontal Programme Committee to the Medical Education Planning Committee was that the methods of evaluation seemed "loose" as attitudes were difficult to measure. The solution was that students would need "continued assessment."[68] Finally, by the end of Phase I, curriculum planners hoped to develop the following attitude characteristics: to feel familiar with health sciences facilities, to understand what her role is as a health professional, and to feel "security in the knowledge that he is responsible for his own education."[69]

The importance of training students who "know themselves" required various methods of instruction. For example, problem statements for the PBL method included questions such as: "What is the relationship between health research at McMaster and patients receiving medical care in Hamilton?"[70] Students would need to be self-learning, interacting with patients throughout their time in the program, developing clinical skills and good attitudes: "Medical students will confront problem-statements through interaction with patients, their families, and communities under the guidance of a practitioner who embodies the goals of the Horizontal Programme."[71] Assignments included grand rounds where students would present a case that exemplifies the problem for consideration and they would engage their peers in small group discussion. There were also activities to help students develop "a greater understanding of their own feelings and their interaction with others."[72] Students were given a range of experiences interviewing patients who had been selected for their different personalities, presentation of symptoms, and so on. Students learned techniques of listening to patients and came to understand the range of emotions they and their patients would encounter in the clinic. This objective was tied into the responsibility of graduates to understand the doctor-patient relationship.[73]

In addition to learning their own emotional limitations, students were also expected to continue to develop their self-directed learning skills for beyond graduation. There was an elective component to the horizontal program. The focus of this requirement was *scholarly* development in research or clinical work. Students were given two six-week periods during their program to learn more about an aspect of medicine of their choosing, again being encouraged to become self-learners but also expected to learn the importance of being clinicians who were also tied to research. Options varied from year to year but included electives in clinical epidemiology, laboratory sciences, or mathematics in medicine, which was about biometrics: "Emphasis will be placed upon understanding the basic approach and not upon arithmetic or formulae." This latter course ran throughout the three phases of the program. The electives provided an opportunity for students to cultivate more interest in the basic sciences and their relevance to the curriculum and clinical practice.[74]

The goal of the horizontal program was to have students ready to undertake their clerkship. The clerkship emphasized that "the link between 'clinical work' and 'basic science' must be constant, direct and meaningful,"[75] which required that students "integrate the earlier 'systems approach' to human biology in its widest sense, into a holistic concept of the patient, his family, his society and his community."[76] The real emphasis was on clinical work and developing "clinical problem-solving" while being able to understand the responsibilities of medicine.[77]

The horizontal program was unique to McMaster in its structure and design, but it met resistance from faculty and students alike. The main skills that were featured in the learning units of the horizontal program were later incorporated into the other phases of the program. For example, in *Progress Report: Horizontal Programme 1971–1972,* clinical interviewing later became part of Phase II.[78] The integration of socio-cultural, ethical, and legal aspects of medical work were brought into Phase III.[79] This report also stated: "It would appear that there really is not a horizontal programme as a unitary phenomenon in our curriculum and that there is no need for such a programme ... By proper integration into the planning of each phase there might be minimization of the 'tacked-on' quality of the horizontal experiences."[80] By the end of 1972, the review of the program listed a number of changes, including renaming the program as the Clinical Skills Program because "Horizontal seems to have outlived its usefulness."[81] Along with this name change, information about health care delivery was included in Phase IV, which left "the remaining objectives of the Horizontal Programme [to] deal mostly with the acquisition of clinical skills, exposure and responsibility."[82]

The horizontal program was about learning "how" to doctor, what ethical and professional duties would be required of graduating physicians. The Education Committee at McMaster hoped students would graduate with "the ability to discern problems and potential problems relevant to his [*sic*] activities in medicine"; "the ability to approach and define the solution of problems relevant to medicine, the patient, his family and the community, by relating back to basic mechanisms"; "[the] ability to seek out and to make effective use of the information and resources required to make decisions and solve problems relevant to his continuing education"; "a critical approach to the assessment of research, diagnosis, prevention and treatment of medical problems"; as well as skills associated with competent examination.[83]

The Tutor System: Responsibilizing Students

I have discussed how the McMaster program was structured so as to ensure that the individual student would become a biological problem-solver in the clinic and a self-learner with regard to keeping up with new information. The horizontal program also taught students that a physician had ethical responsibilities to patients, to herself, and to the community, and that it was imperative that students learn to integrate these duties into their practices. These duties were fundamental to becoming a member of the profession of medicine. Through a Foucauldian analysis of disciplinary power, hierarchical observation, and self-correction, I explained that the program's tactics were appropriate for this form of training. I now explain the tutor system at McMaster as the technique that integrated the core organizing principles, the physical space, and the instruments of evaluation that linked lifelong learners with biomedical problem-solvers. I employ the concept of responsibilization to show how the tutorial system individualized students in order to target their reasoning and judgment, all in the name of changing medical practice and ameliorating clinical judgments. I argue that the disciplinary tactics of PBL resulted in the responsibilization of student subjectivity.

The concept of responsibilization was first coined in sociological and criminological research that examined the ways in which responsibility for crime control was shifted from the state to the individual (O'Malley 1992, 259). These crime control strategies aimed to individualize people who committed crimes and to enlist different organizations to take an active role in the reduction of crime and, more specifically, of the opportunities for people to engage in it. Garland (2001, 124) refers to these measures as responsibilization strategies: they involve "a way of thinking and a variety of techniques designed to change the manner in which" individuals act. In his research, Garland examines the role of neighbourhood watch, which encourages property owners to take responsibility for crime reduction by taking such precautions as locking their doors to prevent people from committing crimes of opportunity. When it comes to improving medical practice through the reform of medical education, individual practitioners become responsible for improving medical care by using information from biomedical sciences – the best available evidence – in their practice. The new program at McMaster conceived of the new student as being a self-learner who had a social obligation to keep up with new information beyond graduation.

The tutoring program at McMaster was guided by various pedagogical principles. The first was underpinned by the expectation that "medical students [would] be graduate students with major responsibility for their own education." And this, in turn, relied on the assumption that "learning requires searching and self-organizing activity devoted to comprehension."[84] Learning was defined as "seeing the essence of problems and utilizing all the resources of the university, living or otherwise, to understand the problem and answer related questions."[85] This reflected a commitment to the link between the clinic and biological and medical sciences. Learning, however, also meant constant self-improvement, which PBL was well-suited to facilitate: "Such a format permits each staff member to learn from his colleagues and by so doing to indicate to students that a constant process of learning occurs and that degrees of expertness are relative."[86] The tutor system was styled in such a way that students would be tutored by non-experts, so that their clinical judgments would be evaluated not just on their accuracy or expertise regarding the content of medical science information but also on how they think through the problem and the steps they take to solve it.

This format meant that students needed to learn how to evaluate themselves.

The goal of the tutor system was to produce students who had "the ability to seek out and to make effective use of the information and resources required to make decisions and solve problems relevant to [their] continuing education."[87] To achieve these goals, the medical program offered a number of different roles to make the tutoring component a success. In response to confusion over what tutors actually do, Sackett wrote a document that spelled out the roles of the different members of the program.[88] Each department in the program consisted of a resource person, a unit chair, a tutor, and the students. The resource person was meant to function as a learning resource for students. They were assigned by a unit chair and, "on demand," would organize an event at which to meet with students. Resource persons were specialists in a given problem and, under the PBL model, they could meet with small groups for discussions.[89] The unit chair determined the objectives of each unit in the medical curriculum and set the criteria for evaluation. There was also the usual expectation that the chair would be responsible for program leadership and administration.[90]

In *Governing Morals,* Alan Hunt (1999, 223) applauds the heuristic usefulness of the concept of responsibilization: "[It] catches the duality of responsibility for the self and for others by drawing attention to the active components of many discourses that assign responsibility to specific categories of agents as is exemplified in the slogan: 'Only you can stop drinking and driving,' which individualizes the responsible driver." The tutor system was designed to instill the dual responsibility of the student's being responsible not only for his own learning but also for the care of others. The responsibilities of the faculty tutor were originally conceived as "helping his individual students, separately and collectively as a small group, to organize their approach to each problem; helping them to seek information which is relevant; helping them to become familiar with the resources of the College of Health Sciences, appropriate resources elsewhere in the university and elsewhere in the community."[91] Later, Sackett amended this statement in its practical application, which also included an element of evaluation and that, later, would become the topic of much debate among the faculty on the education committee. The tutor ought to understand the abilities of the students and their learning objectives and make sure they develop the necessary program knowledge and problem-solving skills. In order to cultivate their learning, the tutor also needed to understand what "other students, health science professionals, the university and the community expect of the medical students."[92] Tutors should also motivate students to learn, know the program objectives and the learning resources available, and evaluate the student's success "in order to further effective methods of self-learning and problem-solving."[93] The tutor was a first point of contact for students who became stuck on problems and was to help them find the right resources.[94] It was evident from this conception of the role of the tutor that she or he was primarily responsible for supervising and evaluating the student's development of self-learning techniques.

The role of the student entailed satisfying all instructional objectives, including assuming "a high degree of responsibility for his education, characterized by: honesty, effective self-learning, biomedical problem-solving, effective interaction with others, [and] setting of goals relevant to personal and community objectives."[95] Students were also required to pursue at least one interest beyond the curriculum units and to provide constructive feedback to the program chairs regarding curriculum development.[96] The student was responsible not only for recognizing that learning was her personal responsibility but also for seeking out individual projects to increase her self-learning skills. Given that "responsibilization refers to a form of governing that discursively imposes specific responsibilities on individuals relating to their own conduct or that of another for whom they are presented as being responsible" (Hunt 2003, 187), being a student meant recognizing and acting on the responsibility to be a self-learner. It was also important for students to provide feedback to the program. While during its early years this was done to improve the program, it also functioned to get students to think about how the program was or was not meeting their personal learning objectives. To para-phrase Hunt (1999, 30), the "participatory responsibilities" of the physician in learning and developing biomedical reasoning and problem-solving skills, evaluating good and bad evidence, and keeping up with the literature were central to the tutorial tech-nique. The tutors were agents of regulation insofar as their role was to train new physicians according to the pedagogical prin-ciples and objectives of the new curriculum.

There was much debate about the tutor system during these early program years. For example, Sackett suggested that tutorial sessions begin only after a tutor completed tutor training, and after the unit chair and planners wrote good problems for the stu-dents. Students were given five problems for each week of a learn-ing unit.[97] Tutors were encouraged to meet with the chair prior to each tutoring session in order to make sure they were on the same page about how to run tutoring sessions, how to go over "key ingredients" of the biomedical problem, how to locate the uni-versal and specific concepts the student should seek out, and how to synthesize them into a solution.[98] Once tutors met with their students and had gone over each of their roles as well as the objec-tives of the unit and horizontal program, then problems were dis-tributed to all students.[99] Tutors met with their assigned students once every four to seven days for half an hour to an hour and a half. Prior to each meeting, students handed in written work, and, during meetings, the tutor critiqued and assessed that work.[100] If the work was not adequate, the student would be expected to redo it and the tutor would be expected to help her find the appropri-ate self-learning aids and resources.[101]

In May 1971, Dr. Adsett prepared a monograph on the role of the tutor, and this was distributed to faculty. He agreed with ear-lier iterations of the roles of unit chairs and tutors, whereby the unit planner was expected to provide the tutor with the objectives of each unit, the problems and materials, without which the tutor would have too much responsibility for planning. In his mono-graph, Adsett defines the tutorial session as follows: "The tuto-rial must be a working session where the students have utilized learning resources on their own and then come to the tutorial prepared to engage in discussion of a problem, how they have approached it and what difficulties they had with it, including the expression of their own ideas and interests."[102]

The role of the tutor was specified as "generalist," as her main asset was "having a general knowledge and experience about medicine" and her primary purpose was to "teach self learning and problem solving techniques."[103] The other characteristics that Adsett mentioned included having a general understanding of small group dynamics, having sufficient self-confidence, and having the support from other faculty so that she could guide the student in her own learning. In addition to having an awareness of biological and educational functions, the tutor was expected to have enough understanding of the social and behavioural aspects of medicine to incorporate the horizontal objectives into the tutorial sessions where appropriate. The tutor was also expected "to evaluate the student in conjunction with the student's own self-evaluation, and in turn tolerate the student's evaluation of himself [*sic*] as a tutor."[104] As for the evaluation process: "The tutor focuses on how the student collects data, analysizes [*sic*] it and reports it rather than on specific content. The tutor has an opportunity for an on-going evaluation of the student's problem solving skills and his attitudes which is a by-product of what goes on in the interaction in the group."[105] There was less emphasis on knowing the content or "getting it right" and more on the student's ability to reason through the problem presented in the sessions.

Given the "newness" of McMaster's pedagogy, students, like faculty, had some difficulty understanding what was expected of them in the tutorial sessions. Adsett proposed solving these issues by training tutors in the "art" of tutoring, regularly meeting with unit chairs, tape-recording tutorials for later review, and educating students about what a tutoring session was supposed to be (i.e., students were to work on their own and then discuss their findings with their tutor). As a result of the tutorial system being one of "non-experts," individual students had to become what Erickson and Doyle (2003, 114) might call "their own policy makers, charting principled courses of action that exhibit their capacity for self-improvement in self-controlled ways." Contrary to other models of medical education, the tutor system was not intended to be competitive (which is how students originally treated it) but, rather, an opportunity to learn from each other.[106]

Evaluations of students in the program were targeted around the achievement of its objectives and aimed to test student progress and competence. Interestingly, the first objective was to "help students to evaluate their own achievement in understanding and learning."[107] Under responsibilizing programs, individuals are "held to the responsible standards established by the institutions concerned" (Erickson and Doyle 2003, 114). In the institutional context of the McMaster medical school, evaluation was a major topic of concern. Along with the effect of the PBL tutorial method on medical curricula, new measures of evaluation were devised to be integrated into the new program. The Education Committee at McMaster sought to evaluate small group work and individual student performance in ways that took into account student "motivation, curiosity, initiation, depth of understanding, and attitudes and ethics."[108] This new model presented challenges with regard to creating satisfactory and effective instruments of evaluation, which led to disagreement among faculty. According to the meeting minutes of January 1971:

> Although the [Education] Committee agreed that the tutor should act as a guide to problem solving and not as a teacher, there was disagreement over his role as an evaluator. Dr. Anderson felt that the tutor should compile relevant data from all available sources, in order to arrive at a comprehensive evaluation. Dr. Sackett, on the other hand, felt that the tutor should be capable enough to evaluate a student's technique of gathering evidence in his approach to solving biological problems.[109]

There was conflict between two perspectives: whether tutors were to act as a learning resource to help students "become efficient self-learners,"[110] which might imply that "to be most effective, tutorials must have a methodology as opposed to being a general 'rap' session,"[111] or whether tutors were also meant to assess the student's self-learning as it developed. In the program review student evaluation remained a large concern with the tutor system: "There is residual concern on the part of some faculty regarding the descriptive, non-quantitative method of reporting progress."[112] The usual quantification of progress would have been numeric grades, but the tutorial system was designed to be more emergent than strictly right or wrong. When students made mistakes, they were responsible for correcting themselves. This method was meant to prepare the student for practice in clinical care, where it was necessary that mistakes result in self-improvement.

Prior to the accreditation visit,[113] the McMaster medical school invited a team of physicians from American universities to evaluate its program, its objectives, its new curriculum, and its pedagogy (i.e., PBL) from May 4 to May 6, 1971. There were a number of issues in the pre-accreditation report submitted by Hilliard Jason. First and foremost, students had difficulties adapting to the new program format, which centred on self-learning. By the spring session of first year, only half of the students reported that they were able to take advantage of the freedoms offered by the program. According to the report, "the students also estimate that substantially less than half of the faculty are fully understanding of and able to function well in the McMaster program," which signalled an ongoing need for better orientation of faculty and staff, and this was cited as a major issue.[114] The report also cited communication between units as a major issue, as well as mentioning that there were communication issues between part-time faculty (who were teaching in Phase IV) and full-time faculty (who had taught in earlier phases of the program).[115] The self-learning format was applauded but it was also criticized. Students had the flexibility to develop their own learning style, thanks to the unscheduled time that was supposed to enable them to become self-directed learners. But this ended up being a major problem because there were only five weeks allotted for each of the topics in Phase III, and these were not tested based on the needs of the students.[116]

The report also stated that the McMaster program needed an "improved evaluation system."[117] Despite the fact that evaluation remained a topic of concern for the faculty prior to the review, the report also referred to the program's format as one of its greatest assets:[118] "the purpose of the tutorial was not the dispensing of information (a posture toward which experts are very prone to move), but rather, it should be a forum in which the student's general progress is assessed, his learning procedures are reviewed, and his growth is facilitated."[119] With regard to evaluation: "The main problem with the evaluation system is that it does not exist."[120] The visit was positive with regard to the clarity of the instructional objectives, but there was much work to do to improve the evaluation of self-learners. If the content of the program was not as high a priority as were problem-solving and self-learning skills, the tutorial system was in need of further work.

Responsibilization individualizes as it targets the thoughts and actions that individuals take to better themselves. And this is observed by examining how programs of conduct are "installed" in institutions. McMaster's medical school curriculum sought to better the practice of medicine by installing a new, reformed method of medical education – PBL. Hunt (2003, 172) suggests understanding responsibilization as an ethic as it does not rely purely on the moral judgment of others:

> An ethical self-governance refers to the significant consequence of responsibilization, namely, the requirement that individuals seek out and fashion an ethical life for themselves. This requirement does not impose prescriptions about the correct conduct of that life. It only demands that life be conducted reflexively, or that the individual be capable of advancing some justification of the choices made.

The student was the individual object of the curriculum, the one who had been given a host of new responsibilities: to judge based on the best biomedical information, to solve clinical problems by using science, and, most important, to become a self-learner and to be motivated to improve her knowledge (a skill she could use to "keep up" with emerging medical information). The adequacy of the student's ability to retain information was secondary to her ability to reflect on her own learning and to seek evidence for herself. The tutorial format required that students learn to develop these skills and evaluate and correct themselves. The disagreement among faculty about evaluation signals that the ultimate objective of training students to perform these tasks and to recognize and develop their duties to these objectives was paramount to curriculum outcomes. The objectives required criteria for and instruments of evaluation to ensure that the curriculum was indeed effective, that students were being trained to perform these skills. Beyond graduation, the performance of these skills was intended to resolve the problems of clinical practice. Reforming medical education meant new methods of training physicians to have better judgment. It meant installing a program of conduct that individualized physicians to the point at which they were able to see that attaining this judgment was a responsibility they had to themselves as well as to others.

Enduring Responsibilities, Maintaining Competence: Continuing Medical Education in Canada

The fundamental principle of becoming a self-directed learner was that it would be a lifelong career commitment. This section examines the McMaster curriculum's effect on continuing medical education in Canada. In the 1960s, the

> Report of the Panel on the General Professional Education of the Physician and College Preparation for Medicine [was] ... sponsored by the Association of American Medical Colleges. This report made many recommendations for changes in medical education, such as promoting independent learning and problem solving, reducing lecture hours, reducing scheduled time, and evaluating the ability to learn independently. (Barrows 1996, 4)

The solution to the link between information and practice was the reform of the medical curriculum, but how could physicians be held responsible for keeping up these duties after graduation? New programs emerged to ensure that students were maintaining their skills, keeping up to date with new information about the effectiveness of emerging medical and therapeutic interventions. Self-directed learning became a tenet of continuing medical education.

The Royal College of Physicians and Surgeons of Canada (RCPSC) is primarily responsible for accrediting residency programs in Canada, in addition to holding medical examinations and assessing the links between education and medical practice in the seventeen programs across the nation. Alongside discussions about reforming medical education in the 1980s, this organization also began to rethink the competence of physicians, seeing it as being linked to their ability to read medical literature and to integrate the best evidence into their practices. In November 1988, the RCPSC held the Workshop on Maintenance of Competence. The list of invited attendees included participants from the provincial licensing authorities, the Canadian Medical Association, and the Canadian Federation of Provincial Colleges, among other regulatory bodies of medicine and medical education. The objective of this meeting was "to develop general policies and specific recommendations for a maintenance of competence system for the specialists of [the RCPSC].[121] There were a number of task forces that were asked to assess the problems physicians had with keeping up to date in various areas. One of the task forces (Task Force 7) was led by Dr. Brian Haynes from McMaster University. His team focused on what was termed "Journals and Written Materials, Including Use of Literatures," and it homed in on the following question: "Should journal reading and other written material be part of a maintenance of competence system? If yes, what should be the system to ensure suitable credit? Should there be extra credit for owning a personal computer and doing literature searches, e.g., Medline?"[122] The critical appraisal method from McMaster would come to guide improvements in the continuing education course.

In July 1991, the RCPSC launched its first initiative to resolve this problem: "Maintenance of Competence (MOCOMP) Pilot Program: An Information Guide for Specialists." The guide for physicians to sign up for the pilot project was introduced with the epigraph:

Rapid change is one of the most striking features of our time. Medical science and technology, the socio-demographic, political and economic structure of our country, even basic tenets of biomedical ethics, are in perpetual ferment. A large part of medical knowledge we possess at the end of our apprenticeship in medical training has become obsolete within 10 years. No specialist can remain competent without taking energetic steps to keep in touch with the growing edge of the specialty.[123]

The program was a response to the need to reform medical education and to keep physicians up to date on the newest information. The pilot project aimed to recruit physicians as a test of its main objective, which was to revise the "curriculum of CME [continuing medical education] which, if followed, [would] assist the physician to keep abreast of advances in medicine."[124] The publications cited the reasons for changing the CME programs: "We live in a time when the public wants to participate in clinical decisions and wants to be informed about their health problems. This new environment can provide job satisfaction for the well-informed specialist, but can be stressful to those who are not keeping up to date."[125] In a published recruitment notice, the October 1991 MOCOMP Bulletin stressed the need for physicians to maintain their self-directed and problem-based learning and to practise relevant skill sets. The program materials included problem-based learning activities.[126]

These programs were installed by regulatory institutions for the purposes of resolving the problematized aspects of clinical care. As evidence that this program targeted clinical judgments, I briefly discuss the February 1994 RCPSC workshop titled "Maintenance of Competence/Monitoring of Performance," which was offered in Quebec by the Federation of Medical Licensing Authorities of Canada (FMLAC). This workshop was attended by FMLAC executives, representatives from nine out of ten provincial colleges of physicians and surgeons, the Medical Council of Canada, the RCPSC, the CMA, the College of Family Physicians, and an invited guest from the National Board of Medical Examiners of the United States.[127] Its purpose was "to identify performance problems in physicians and to propose a system of maintenance of competence/monitoring of performance."[128] Subsequent goals included specifying the role of provincial authorities in regulating physician competence.[129]

Although those in attendance understood "the Mission of the licensing authorities [as] ... protect[ing] the public by guaranteeing that physicians are competent when they enter practice and that their performance throughout their professional lives continues to meet the needs and expectations of society,"[130] it was only just prior to this workshop that a national licensing exam was established, and many members of the workshop thought this was the time to enforce a standard for maintaining practice. The workshop defined the physician's knowledge as "information stored in the physician's mind"; it defined competence as one's "ability to appropriately apply knowledge"; and it defined performance as the doctor's ability to translate competence into action to care for a patient.[131] This last definition is reminiscent of the PBL method, which attempts to facilitate the physician's ability to recall and apply medical facts in the clinic. Information had to be appropriately translated into practice. Ideally, this translation happened through the physician's judgment: taking what she knew (which meant that she ought to be up to speed on the best practices) and putting it to work to improve patient care.

There was discussion about how to assess physicians, which workshop participants decided meant asking whether physicians knew the right things, whether they could apply them, and whether they actually did so.[132] The licensing authorities had to have a clear understanding of what was the correct answer to these questions, and clinical practice guidelines were important for understanding the regulatory powers of the colleges. One of the four major problems identified with physician performance included deficient management of care, which was defined as the tendency for clinical performance to "decay over time." The solution proposed by the workshop attendees involved the use of clinical practice guidelines: "The proposed ideal system presented by this group included guidelines to determine appropriate management of care."[133] The working group stated that physicians are "accountable" and that their "structure, process and outcome should be monitored" through various types of "critical appraisal."[134] The licensing authorities were identified as being responsible for regulating physician judgments: "The licensing authority would be responsible for monitoring, identification and decision-making regarding individual physicians who had problems in clinical performance."[135] The colleges already had established processes for dealing with complaints regarding deficient management of care.[136]

The specific formulation of the physician as the individual responsible for the improvement of bedside care, for the elimination of the problems of clinical practice, gave way to a host of responsibilization strategies that were installed at the site of medical education. The summary report from the accreditation visit to McMaster's new program in 1972 states that its "curriculum is innovative and probably more effective in stressing the responsibility of the student for his [sic] own education than any other model in North America."[137] As a result, PBL continued to be touted as the best way to train clinicians to learn to read and integrate new knowledge into their clinical practices. One of the first examples of the primacy of PBL may be found in an article in *Academic Medicine* written by Vernon and Blake. They performs a meta-analysis of all the studies that compare PBL to other curricula and what they found confirmed the "superiority of the PBL approach" (Vernon and Blake 1993, 550) to medical training. They concluded that PBL remains the best method to train physicians to use biomedical information and to learn biomedical problem solving.

The McMaster program provides a case study that illuminates the link between problematization and a program of conduct. Its program relied on techniques that train physicians to become self-motivated and lifelong learners. This notion also underpins other programs of conduct, such as the MOCOMP program at the RCPSC. There is an emphasis on individualizing clinicians to help them keep up with new information, and this requires the creation of programs that can provide ongoing training. The big questions of evaluating self-learning, however, are relocated to regulatory mechanisms, the provincial licensing colleges being tasked with the ongoing evaluation of these professional duties to keep up. Now that I have explained both the material relations that organized the new model of medical training and the techniques that responsibilized physicians, I turn to examining the use of the clinical practice guideline, how it emerged, and its links with EBM, the responsibility to keep up, and disciplinary regulation.

4

Technologies of Regulation: Clinical Practice Guidelines and the Effects of Normalization

THE CASE STUDY of the McMaster University medical program demonstrates that the solution to the various problematizations of clinical practice was the reform of medical education. By combining a new science of clinical epidemiology with new spaces, students learn to integrate different professional knowledges into their practice. Further, the installation of a new curriculum in medical education is predicated on an ideal-typical student – the self-learner. The disciplinary tactics of the problem-based learning model constitute the student as responsible for not only using evidence but also for keeping up with it. The tutor system incites students to seek out information to biomedical problems, thus training them to become self-motivated learners. The rationale for this goal is the need to teach students how to assess evidence and then continue their own learning beyond graduation. Whether or not students were doing this was another problem – not only for their evaluation during medical school but also once they joined the profession. Continuing medical education programs were designed in collaboration with the Royal College of Physicians and Surgeons of Canada to facilitate the skills of critical appraisal and keeping up. CME came to be regulated, however, by each provincial licensing jurisdiction. The question of who would monitor the responsibilized physician was answered by placing that role within the jurisdiction of the provincial colleges. This chapter discusses the role that the colleges play with regard to keeping up, specifically in relation to the regulatory procedures that are set up to monitor and judge the physician's good use of evidence in practice.

Here I spell out the force relations that regulate and normalize clinical judgment. Following Foucault (2000, 340), I show how the specificity of power relations exists in their exercise: power is a mode of action that acts on the actions of subjects. The provincial colleges assume the authority to discipline and regulate the actions of practising physicians. I show how the force relation termed "normalization" played a role in regulating the profession of medicine and the lifelong learner post-graduation. The effects of this strategy, however, produce results that are considered failures of the evidence-based medicine training program, which holds that physicians ought to defer to guidelines rather than to assess the evidence. This chapter's argument is necessary to establish the effects of the dispositif: the success of the normalization of clinical judgment and its failure to meet the imagined goal of evidence-based judgment. Once readers understand the effects and the nature of what force relations normalize, I go on, in the final chapter, to explain why EBM is able to keep going despite its failures.

Problematizing Keeping Up

By the 1990s, there was so much evidence that clinical practice guidelines became a source of attention. Additionally, the social context of an economic recession brought about concerns regarding the growing cost of medical care. For example, Schoenbaum (1993) suggested a way of measuring the outcomes of health care by developing guidelines that could improve the economic costs of medical care. If health care could decrease the number of medical procedures, it could reduce the costs of care; and if physicians made correct decisions more frequently, they would not order inappropriate tests or provide unnecessary and costly care. Proponents of evidence-based medicine, particularly Sackett and colleagues, refute the claim that EBM was introduced to cut the cost of care. In fact, they contend the opposite: improved health care will ultimately result in higher costs (Sackett et al. 2000, 18).

So if claims about EBM were not related to a changing economic or managerial landscape, what discursive principles underpinned an emerging focus on clinical practice guidelines (and later evidence-based CPGs) throughout the 1980s and 1990s? David Eddy explains that the shift in the focus of the medical literature went from medical authority, the conventional assumption that "doctors know best," to questions about the credibility of clinical judgments. He argues that using evidence in medical practice could respond to both questions about economic cost and questions about reported variations in care (Eddy 1993, 521–23). In addition to questions about practice variation, the medical school reforms that had been under way throughout the 1970s led to a variety of important issues in clinical epidemiology. For example, the first edition of Fletcher, Fletcher, and Wagner's (1982, 217) textbook on teaching clinical epidemiology to medical students argues that students should learn to critically analyze and appraise the evidence they encounter in medical journals in order to make decisions about which data and evidence are valid and relevant. This is consistent with the reforms made to the McMaster program. By the publication of the third edition of their textbook in 1996, Fletcher, Fletcher, and Wagner (1996, 266) advocate that physicians use practice guidelines that are developed through EBM. While it is important to continue questioning guidelines on the basis of inclusivity for all populations and the most accurate and up-to-date medical research, the use of guidelines, they argue, improves the health outcomes of patients.

There was a shift in Fletcher, Fletcher, and Wagner's position on student education and training. First, they argued for the importance of teaching the skills required for the critical analysis of evidence in medical education, which was in line with their epidemiologic principles of "counting" the best evidence in clinical practice. In the third edition of their book, however, they argue for a different convention in medical education, one that may appear antithetical to the stated aims of clinical epidemiology – the move towards practice guidelines. Practice guidelines shift the physician's analysis of the evidence to the guideline creators, and, ideally, guidelines lay out a course of action appropriate to clinical situations. The reformulation of the goals of clinical epidemiology to EBM demonstrates the normative dimension of this problematization: keeping up with the literature was onerous despite the fact that, under newly institutionalized medical training, it was the physician's responsibility to do so. The correction of this new problem relied on existing technologies of regulation that were repurposed to monitor the activities of physicians, specifically judgments based on the best evidence.

After the appearance of EBM in the literature conversations about practice guidelines became more predominant. EBM would come to provide the rationale for CPGs as a strategic intervention at the level of individual judgment, and Canada's provincial medical colleges are now playing an active role in deploying this technology to determine the difference between good and poor medical judgments. To advance this claim, I first spell out the link between EBM (its appearance and its normalization of risk) and CPGs as a strategy to improve health care at the level of individual judgments. Next, I discuss the Canadian context under which a new partnership between government and medical regulation came to create a CPG repository for practising physicians. Then, I provide evidence to show that provincial colleges are endorsing CPGs and using them as a way to discipline physicians. I do this by constructing a database of disciplinary decisions taken from every English-speaking provincial medical college across Canada. The chapter concludes by looking at the ontology of clinical judgment when it is normalized by disciplinary sanctions.

Normalizing Risk: The Relations of Discourse

Foucault's (1979, 136–38) analytic for "discipline" spells out the ways that, in systems of punishment, the individualized body comes to be the target and effect of power; the body is rendered intelligible by various discourses, such as psychiatry or education, as a problematic object that could be improved and transformed. In the prison or asylum, confinement was one of the main tactics whereby relations of power could act on subjects. For physicians, however, the target and effect of disciplinary action is not the body, and it is not my intention to show that practitioners are confined. Instead, what was rendered intelligible by the discourses of medicine and education was clinical judgment. With regard to medical regulation in Canada, Foucault is helpful in that he enables us to see how individual judgments come to be normalized through a system of professional disciplinary action that, to paraphrase him, seeks to construct judgments as problematic should they depart from what is deemed correct behaviour (178).

According to Foucault's (1979, 158) analysis of punishment, disciplinary tactics are applied so that the subject reaches a required level of aptitude. Tactics are defined as "the art of constructing, with located bodies, coded activities and trained aptitudes, mechanisms in which the product of the various forces is increased by their calculated combination" (167). In EBM, the site of these relations is the clinician's judgment insofar as CPGs aim to improve physician decision-making behaviours. The decision-making activities of medicine are coded and regulated in provincial colleges and professional policies for correct procedure. The aptitudes of physicians are assessed in disciplinary hearings, which I discuss later on.

EBM endorses CPGs as strategies for changing clinician behaviour (Guyatt, Haynes, et al. 2008). Guidelines can allow physicians to make clinical decisions based on "medically relevant" evidence, which regulates the assessment of risk (Guyatt, Haynes, et al. 2008, 14). In their practices, physicians are to interpret a symptom using "clinical expertise" and CPGs. When they are used to regulate physicians' activities, CPGs can be understood as programs of disciplinary conduct. To paraphrase Foucault (2003, 252), that provincial medical colleges use evidence-based CPGs to evaluate clinical judgments is a "codifying effect" of EBM. CPGs are codes of conduct, general rules to be applied in particular cases. CPGs rule in and rule out what clinical or paraclinical evidence is relevant to diagnosis, treatment, and/or medical interventions (e.g., further tests, therapies, or medical procedures) in a variety of diseases, and they render individual judgments visible as a target of intervention and amelioration.

In Foucault's analytic of regulation, individual cases are deemed problematic by being observed in an institutional context. The medical community's endorsement of CPGs indicates that there is an interest in normalizing good judgments in medical practice (also indicated by the alternate term "best practices"). Foucault (1979, 181) explains that normalizing judgments occurs through the observation of conduct, which is then graded in a distribution – a procedure that differentiates individual "cases" from the norm or rule for correct conduct. CPGs normalize clinical judgments in relation to that which is recommended as a course of action. CPGs are "rules" insofar as they aim to organize human activity in the clinic by differentiating between good and bad judgments. EBM provides a knowledge base, or rationale, for justifying regulatory interventions in the clinic.

Guidelines are not a new phenomenon in medical practice. The first publications of recommendations for clinical practice appeared in the United States as early as 1931 (Weisz et al. 2007, 702). Weisz and colleagues argue that CPGs represent "a change in the method of regulating the quality of medical practice" (692). Guidelines began to appear more regularly by the 1980s, when there was an effort to organize "a rapidly expanding and heterogeneous medical domain" (ibid.). Weisz and colleagues explain that the regulation of medical practice was undergirded by expertise and conventionalism up until the 1970s, with the authority of medical knowledge providing the backbone for public trust in clinical care (693). Throughout the 1970s and 1980s, there was a shift away from relying on the "opinions of experts": "In contrast, the regulation of quality now explicitly targets medical practice itself by attempting to modify physicians' behavior" (693). My research shows that questioning medical authority was but one problematization of clinical practice, and I present an alternate explanation for the influence of CPGs on medical practice. The problematization of clinical judgment in combination with the emerging responsibilization of individual practitioners to keep up with new information provided the justification for a new professional technology of regulation – the CPG – to regulate the clinic.

On the heels of the first EBM statements, Grimshaw and Russell (1993, 1317), two supporters of EBM, published a paper that sought to test whether guidelines that are evidence-based are effective with regard to the outcomes of care. They argue that, although the clinical significance of their findings may be questionable, "explicit guidelines do improve clinical practice, in the context of rigorous evaluations" (1321). Evaluations function as checks and balances to test the effects of guidelines and their implementation strategies. The evaluation procedure points to areas where physicians are not employing guidelines in their practice, and it serves to encourage strategies for implementation so as to bring clinical care into what is considered best practice.

Later, in 2004, Grimshaw and colleagues published a health technology assessment report that they prepared for the National Health Service, Department of Research and Development Health Technology Assessment Programme, in the United Kingdom. This document reports on a systematic review of guideline development and implementation strategies. It concludes that "the majority of interventions observed modest to moderate improvements in care" (iii), and that "there is an imperfect evidence base to support decisions about which guideline dissemination and implementation strategies are likely to be efficient under different circumstances" (iv). The report suggests that it is necessary to determine a scientific rationale for implementation strategies and guideline development due to the fact that "there was considerable variation in the observed effects both within and across interventions" (61).

The solutions to the problems of implementation were formulated by two working groups, the GRADE (Grading of Recommendations Assessment, Development and Evaluation) Working Group and the AGREE (Appraisal of Guidelines for Research and Evaluation) Collaboration. GRADE was headed by Guyatt (one of the original EBM working group members), and it continues to be a system for ranking the quality of evidence. The idea behind GRADE is that an objective system can determine whether physicians can be confident about practice recommendations that follow from RCTs or meta-reviews of the literature. The authors justify the need for such an instrument through the example of hormone replacement therapy. In the 1990s, it became common-place for physicians to prescribe hormone therapy to their post-menopausal patients in order to lower the risk of cardiovascular disease. After a decade of research, it was shown that this practice "fail[ed] to reduce cardiovascular risk and may even increase it" (Guyatt, Oxman, et al. 2008, 924). The authors contend that, had there been a system in place for measuring the confidence that one can have in the evidence on which evidence is based, this – and other faulty practices – could have been avoided.

GRADE ranks recommendations to "indicate whether *(a)* the evidence is high quality and the desirable effects clearly outweigh the undesirable effects, or *(b)* there is a close or uncertain balance" (Guyatt, Oxman, et al. 2008, 925). Guideline development, which was meant to reduce problems resulting from practice variation and the integration of the best information into clinical practice, had produced its own problematic consequences. The focus on generating recommendations to normalize clinical practice led to the reproduction of those same problems: How can physicians know whether the best evidence was used or not? GRADE aimed to resolve this problem by categorizing evidence as "strong" and "weak," and by reducing variables such as patient preferences and advice that relied on conventional wisdom or "expertise" (Guyatt, Oxman, et al. 2008, 925).[1] The method of evidence-ranking and appraisal designed by GRADE provided a scientific rationale for clinical intervention. Measuring the outcomes of care, their effectiveness, and the strength of evidence on which general recommendations could be made linked the need to make decisions based on the best available evidence with the need to keep up with new information.

As guideline production became routinized in clinical research,[2] there was an increase in the number of recommendations appearing in the literature. As the Canadian Medical Association (2011, 4) puts it, "multiple conflicting guidelines are being developed by different groups in an uncoordinated way, creating a 'morass.'" If there are multiple recommendations for the same disease, how can physicians know which one is the best, even if there is more than one that meets GRADE criteria? AGREE is an international collaboration that is developing an international grading system for guideline creation: "As the number of published guidelines proliferates, there have been calls for the establishment of internationally recognized standards to improve the development and reporting of clinical guidelines" (Cluzeau and AGREE Collaboration 2003, 18). According to the AGREE group instrument, the quality of the guidelines varies – some are absolute, some are not. Their appraisal method is intended to provide discretionary advice, assessing the process of the guideline's development, but neither the conditions under which the evidence was generated nor the quality of the results is included (ibid.).

With the proliferation of guidelines, practice variation continues to be problematic. EBM requires physicians to use the best evidence in their clinical decision making, and doctors have been responsibilized to keep up with new information. Given that there is *so much* information, however, the impossibility of this task has led to guideline development. There are now multiple guidelines, and practice variation has become a concern. AGREE responds to this by providing a standard for evaluating the process of guideline creation. Practitioners can then know which guidelines not only have the best evidence but also rely on the quality of their development. Where these questions become even more fascinating is where the concerns about practice variation and regulation intersect. I now discuss the Canadian context of guidelines implementation.

Creating a Resource: The Canadian Context

In Canada, guidelines not only seek to normalize clinical practice but also to standardize future outcomes in health care. At the turn of the millennium, the Canadian first ministers of health met to identify problems with health care systems across Canada. While health care and its management are under provincial jurisdiction, the function of this new Health Council of Canada (HCC) was to "monitor and make annual public reports on the implementation of the Accord, particularly its accountability and transparency provisions" (Health Canada 2003). Here I explore the relations that came to organize human activity by examining a governmental and institutional partnership that aimed to intervene in the management of care by creating a CPG database for physicians to use in their practices.

At its conception, the HCC was only mandated to prepare an "annual report to all Canadians, on the health status of Canadians and health outcomes" (Health Canada 2004). The focus of these annual reports was health care system delivery, the idea being to improve the standard of care across Canada and, to some extent, standardize it. As time passed, the HCC reoriented itself towards a new mission – to provide "a more accessible, higher quality, and sustainable health care system" (Health Council of Canada 2011, b). HCC's new mandate also stipulated that it would "let governments and the Canadian public know how progress towards this vision [was] coming along" (2). The HCC's mission and mandate reflected the close relationship between reporting on health care systems improvement and actively initiating projects for the betterment of health care.

The HCC worked in partnership with a number of associations, including the Canadian Medical Association, to meet its new mandate. This relationship not only provided the HCC (2011, 5) with access to medical expertise but also reoriented its focus so that it "place[d] greater emphasis on identifying, reporting and disseminating best practices and innovation in its public reports." These groups would report to both Canadians and to physicians about best practices, using evidence-based research and outcomes. The underlying rationale for communicating with the CMA and disseminating CMA-supported research was to improve the health of Canadians: "The Council considers progress in terms of its overall impact on the health status and health outcomes of Canadians" (6). These communications would inform practitioners of best practices as well as provide recommendations to the government on how to strengthen the health care system through the use of best practice guidelines (10–11). If CPGs could be developed for major illnesses and disseminated to physicians across Canada, this would improve the health of Canadian society. The target of this policy initiative placed the onus of better care on best practice, which translated into improving the decisions of the acting physician rather than into providing greater funding resources or infrastructure support to the provinces. The reasoning was that if judgments could be standardized through CPGs then care would improve.

The HCC formed a collaborative partnership with the CMA to generate research on best practices. This strategy of enlisting expert knowledge from medicine fell in line with the solutions proposed by EBM. To improve care across the country, what was needed was doctors who made similar judgments, and the best judgments would be those based on the best available evidence. They HCC and CMA co-sponsored a joint initiative, the Canadian Clinical Practice Guidelines Summit (the Summit), which was held in November 2011. The Summit was attended by various health care stakeholders, including government ministers, representatives of the provincial colleges, various societies for effective practice, and private health consulting agencies. The Summit's published report states that the goals of the meeting were concerned with "reaching consensus that CPGs deserve attention at the policy level; developing a shared understanding of priorities to improve the overall CPG process; exploring the feasibility of a national CPG strategy" (CMA 2011, 1–2). It notes that one of the obstacles to good care concerns an inability to deal with the production and implementation of knowledge: "This inability to keep pace with current knowledge is one of the reasons for the widening gap between what is considered to be optimal care and the level of care currently provided" (1). Since the Summit, the CMA has created its own repository of guidelines, and individual provincial colleges, such as the CPSO (College of Physicians and Surgeons of Ontario), have endorsed CPGs for their practitioners.

The HCC, the institution and profession of medicine (CMA), and the procedures of EBM (e.g., calculations of the probability for the outcomes of a medical intervention) form complex relations between the knowledge of health care and the means by which the governance of health care seeks to secure the desired ends.

As a technology of EBM, CPGs aim to produce the conditions, in the form of general rules, that would control for national and provincial variation in health care delivery. CPGs have the objective of improving health care and the "health outcomes of Canadians." Solutions to the problems of medicine are derived from medical research and expertise. CPGs assist doctors in their decision making by offering a series of choices that they may follow. These choices, however, have been delimited by the objectives of EBM research and government to improve health outcomes. The guidelines provide a baseline for assessing individual conduct, reproducing the norm regarding what decisions ought to be made and in what ways. Guidelines are meant to keep the freedom of doctors within a "certain range of acceptable conduct." According to the HCC (2012, 2): "When designed and used properly, CPGs – evidence-based recommendations that help health care professionals make appropriate clinical decisions – can, and should, play an important role in the Canadian health care system." The HCC has produced four videos that offer background information on CPGs, and these are freely available to the public on the HCC website.

According the HCC (2012, 3), CPGs can improve Canadian society through better health care:

> There are many benefits to CPGs. They enhance patient quality of care by promoting effective clinical interventions and discouraging ineffective practices. CPGs can also reduce practice variations by helping clinicians across the country to deliver the most evidence-informed care regardless of geography or clinical setting. In addition, CPGs provide standards for the appropriateness of care to which health care providers and health care systems can be held accountable. CPGs may also

contribute to system efficiencies by providing clinicians with information on the most cost-effective practices available.

The HCC also considers knowledge of cost when measuring the efficiency and effectiveness of CPGs. Securing the judgments of individual clinicians in order to control for practice variation also requires an evaluation of cost.

CPGs intervene at the site of individual judgments through relations that structure which courses of action are possible, which is what Nikolas Rose (1993, 298) shows to be a strategy of advanced liberalism: "Advanced liberalism asks whether it is possible to govern ... through the regulated and accountable choices of autonomous agents." For example, Maureen Charlebois, director of clinical adoption at Canada Health Infoway, is quoted in an official CMA document as saying: "This [creating CPGs] isn't about technology, it's about changing [physician] behaviour" (CMA 2011, 7). The objective of CPGs is to reduce practice variation, which requires that the field of possible actions be organized through a calculated set of recommendations that are based on clinical epidemiology research on effectiveness: "In practice, CPGs can range from simple checklists to elaborate decision trees or diagnosis pathways, depending on the type of care, clinical condition, or patient population the guidelines are meant to support" (HCC 2012, 3).

CPGs both disseminate best practices and *implement* them (CMA 2011, 7):

> Health care providers are challenged to stay abreast of continuously emerging clinical research and, as a result, constantly evolving CPGs. Health care providers also must identify the most appropriate CPG from many that are available from a variety of sources. Some key concerns are that CPGs vary widely in terms of their design, the sophistication and rigour of their methodological development, the nature of input of experts and patients, and the influence of special interests. There needs to be repositories of high quality CPGs that clinicians can access efficiently. (HCC 2012, 4)

Studies about "changing physician behaviour, which show that fairly simple interventions can have a large impact on the quality of care" (CMA 2011, 3), are the result of an EBM committed to resolving the problematized aspects of clinical work. These guidelines, however, have the potential to restrict the individual practitioner from implementing his or her own judgment. Indeed, the guidelines are becoming the basis for evaluating individual conduct, and they constrain the doctor's use of the skills associated with critical appraisal and keeping up. It is interesting to note, however, that, according to policy statements, where there are no guidelines it is the doctor's judgment that remains the authority: "Patients should also appreciate that there are many instances when providers will supplement CPG recommendations with their own clinical judgment and expertise to deliver care that is tailored to a patient's specific needs" (HCC 2012, 3). In what follows, I further elucidate this tension between the implementation of guidelines and the responsibility of physicians to employ clinical expertise.

Disciplinary Decisions

In a disciplinary hearing, CPGs that are endorsed by medical colleges or associations may be used as a yardstick for measuring the physician's judgment. In each of Canada's ten provinces, there is a professional college of physicians and surgeons that is responsible for regulating the profession and practice of medicine. One of their legal responsibilities is the privilege to self-regulate and discipline their members. The colleges determine what conduct is good or acceptable and what conduct requires disciplinary action. As an example, the CPSO defines professional misconduct as the "failure to maintain the standard of practice for the profession" (Ontario Regulation 856/93). In legal terms, this is different from the standard of care; however, under federal corporation rights, the colleges have the right to determine what is and is not professional conduct. I now discuss the relationship between college guideline endorsements and medical regulation.

In Canada, physicians are disciplined by medical licensing authorities when they have acted unprofessionally: "Provincial authorities have the ability to police and regulate the quality of medicine through disciplinary action." The profession is made aware of physician misconduct through a complaints process. Each of the provincial medical colleges in Canada has a formal complaints process and a procedure for adjudication: "All complaints of patient negligence, professionalism and sexual abuse are considered serious matters and are usually dealt with by recourse to individual CPS [College of Physicians and Surgeons] regulatory policy" (Alam et al. 2011, E167). According to the Canadian Medical Protective Association (CMPA), from whom the majority of Canadian physicians receive medical malpractice protection, the number of reported medical complaints is decreasing, a fact that is attributed to professional mechanisms that deal with the process. This, in turn, is lowering the number of medical malpractice litigation suits (Canadian Health Services Research Foundation 2006).

In every province, the college of physicians and surgeons has a process in place for dealing with complaints about its licensed members. Patients' complaints are first dealt with by a committee that reviews each complaint individually and either resolves it or refers it on for disciplinary action or tribunal. When complaints are received, physician and patient records are reviewed, occasionally along with patient and physician statements, in order to determine whether a violation of professional conduct has occurred. Complaints may be resolved through actions as simple as, for example, an apology or an order for the physician to take additional education or training. If the complaint is deemed serious enough, it may go on to a hearing, unless the accused physician agrees to cooperate, which means, in some cases, to "plead guilty" and agree to the terms set by the college to ameliorate their professional wrongdoings. A disciplinary decision has many possible outcomes, depending on the province's medical act. For the category of professional misconduct, which is the focus of my investigation, outcomes may include, among other things, suspending or revoking the physician's certificate of registration (i.e., removing her licence to practice), charging a fine, and/or imposing limitations on the physician's practice.

There is an emerging relationship between physician responsibilities and professional regulation. The RCPSC and the Medical Council of Canada have both endorsed Medical Professionalism in the New Millennium: A Physician Charter – a 2002 statement that was issued by the American Board of Internal Medicine, the American College of Physicians, and the European Federation of Internal Medicine. It details a set of professional responsibilities, which, according to the CMPA, play a role in evaluating physician conduct after a complaint has been filed. For example, the CMPA explains that CPGs can play a role in assessing physician conduct. Within the set of professional responsibilities defined by the CMPA, the section titled "Medical Professionalism" spells out the place of practice guidelines in two subsections: "Commitment to the Distribution of Finite Resources" and "Commitment to Maintaining Trust." The former recognizes the physician's commitment to uphold guidelines for cost-effective care, and the latter emphasizes that guidelines are central to the relationship between physicians, patients, and industry. Physicians are expected to participate in the process of self- or professionally led regulation, including "holding each other accountable for their actions" (CMPA 2012). Physicians must respect the rights of the college to regulate its members through the complaints and disciplinary process. Further, the CMPA receives many requests concerning the relevance of CPGs in legal proceedings and complaint processes. Although guidelines are not equivalent to the standard of care as defined within legal proceedings in Canada, they can, through professional mechanisms of regulation, play a role in assessing physician conduct: "Guidelines and statements do not have the force of law, but are influential in defining the appropriate standard of care to which physicians may be held in a legal proceeding *or College complaint*" (CMPA 2014, emphasis added).

In the interest of explaining the effects of EBM and the regulatory technology of guidelines, I built a database of disciplinary decisions from across all English-speaking Canadian medical colleges. Given that the Summit occurred in 2011, I selected a date-range from 2010 to 2016 and collected all disciplinary decision statements that provincial colleges of medicine released to the public. There were 261 statements included in my sample from the following provinces: British Columbia, Alberta, Saskatchewan, Manitoba, Ontario,[3] New Brunswick, Nova Scotia, Prince Edward Island, and Newfoundland and Labrador. These statements were freely available to the public through the college websites, and the information they contain includes a summary of evidence, the basis for the college's decision, and the penalty levied against the accused physician. Allegations include, among many others, contravening the Medical Act, poor record-keeping, the use of improper billing codes, violations of the criminal code, and sexual misconduct. I coded the statements that specifically deemed that the physician was found to have acted "unprofessionally." I then compared the violation to the guidelines that would have been available to the physician given the context of the complaint. I discuss those decisions that determined the physician had behaved unprofessionally in relation to college-endorsed guidelines.

At the time of this writing, it is not a legal requirement for physicians to follow guidelines, but the relationship between college regulation and physician behaviour is changing. According to Foucault (1979, 184), normalization is a productive relation of power insofar as the norm/rule can only standardize as a result of a measurement, which introduces "all the shading of individual difference" between the individual case and the norm. The examination of individual cases, such as a disciplinary committee decision, uses a "normalizing gaze, a surveillance which makes it possible to qualify, to classify, and to punish" (ibid.). Individual cases become analyzable through documentation, which facilitates the classification and normalization of each case within a group (190–91). The group norm is established through the policy or guideline, which acts as the ideal measure of a good decision.

The examination of the individual cases constitutes the individual judgment under scrutiny as an object and effect of power and an effect and object of knowledge (192).

Every college has a list of endorsed guidelines. Not every provincial college, however, stipulates that physicians ought to use the endorsed guidelines to better their practices. To that effect, only the CPSO, CPSS, CPSBC, and CPSA state in their codes of conduct that physicians ought to use guidelines in their practice.[4] I observed that these guidelines are used as a "code" of conduct whereby professional conduct can be classified as misconduct, and tribunals that evaluate disciplinary actions use language similar to that found in the endorsed guidelines. Many decisions do not state that the conduct was measured in relation to the guideline, but it is evident that misconduct is illuminated by the difference between what can be read in the guideline and what is considered inappropriate in (or inappropriately omitted from) a particular practice. The guidelines are used as rules according to which the normalizing judgment of the committee differentiates professional from unprofessional conduct in individual cases. For example, the guideline for Independent Health Facilities for Sleep Medicine, "Clinical Practice Parameters and Facility Standards," states that the college's goal in creating these standards is "to promote activities which will *improve* the level of quality of care by the majority of physicians" (emphasis added). Yet the college also states that guidelines are not meant to replace the physician's judgment: "The parameters and standards are not intended to either replace a physician's clinical judgment or to establish a protocol for all patients with a particular condition. It is understood that ... a particular parameter will rarely be the only appropriate approach to a patient's condition" (CPSO 2013, 1). Guidelines appear to be technologies that are meant to be productive, to facilitate better decision making by rendering the actions of clinicians intelligible, as their recommendations are located at the site of the clinician's judgment: they make recommendations for what the physician should do.

The disciplinary decisions evaluate both procedure and the judgment of clinicians. For example, Dr. Botros (CPSO 2015a) was found to have committed professional misconduct on three counts that relate directly to CPSO-endorsed guidelines regarding sleep medicine. According to the college decision, he failed to maintain the standard of practice with regard to his sleep study interpretation regarding all 22 [complaining] patients. The independent experts retained by the College and Independent Health Facilities, Clinical Practice Parameters and Facility Standards, Sleep Medicine (the Standards) were clear that the sleep medicine physician needed to provide a report of the sleep medicine physician's interpretation of the sleep study data so that the referring physician would know what the diagnosis was and if there was a problem, the recommendation. Dr. Botros's Standard Sleep Study Interpretation form documented neither of these.

I compared this decision statement to the CPSO guideline for sleep medicine, which stipulates that "the interpretation report of a portable monitoring study should include comment on and/ or confirm" a number of details, such as pre- and post-test sleep questionnaires, heart rate abnormalities, suggestions for further investigations and management, and any critically abnormal test results that may need further diagnostic testing (CPSO 2010, 12). Dr. Botros's failing can be seen in direct relation to the kinds of procedures he was meant to follow, such as issuing a report, which were set out in the college-endorsed guideline.

The second infraction listed in the disciplinary decision statement concerns Dr. Botros's failure "to triage all patient referrals as required by the Standards," where the guideline details a number of correct triage procedures (e.g., p. 22). Further, the guideline states: "All referrals must be triaged for appropriateness of testing by a sleep clinician and contain the following: Signature of the physician or surgeon. Demographic data including any medical conditions and medications. Clinical information relevant to the referral. Options for 'Study Only,' 'Consultation,' or 'Both'" (CPSO 2010, 33). This is another example of how the physician's conduct is standardized through the use of CPSO guidelines: when comparing the conduct of the physician to the guideline, the disciplinary committee identified that triage procedures were not followed correctly. This differed from the norm stipulated in the CPG, and thus the conduct was determined to be unprofessional.

The third transgression of the guideline pointed to new concerns: that the judgment of the clinician was unprofessional. Dr. Botros was found to have "allowed two patients to be prescribed CPAP without first being seen by a sleep physician." The guideline states that "the sleep physician requesting PAP titration and subsequently prescribing PAP is required to see and examine the patient and review the sleep study prior to PAP requisition and prescription" (CPSO 2013, 8). The committee's decision moves beyond procedural issues about reporting and communicating with other physicians (which are principles and responsibilities detailed in the Physician Practice Guide [CPSO 2007]), and beyond triage procedures (which include duties spelled out in the Medical Act), and targets the judgment of the clinician. The examination, its specificities, and it recommendations for prescription are made in the guidelines. Although there is no CPSO policy that clearly states that following guidelines is required, it is evident that the CPSO Discipline Committee assesses the cases of physician misconduct in light of these endorsed rules.

The use of endorsed guidelines to normalize conduct can be observed in other provinces as well. The CPSBC makes a distinction between the standard of care and CPGs: standard of care is the minimum standard of practice required by the profession, whereas CPGs are recommendations for courses of action based on the values, principles, and duties of the medical profession, and physicians are expected to use them at their discretion. There were five cases in my sample from British Columbia in which a guideline was used to assess unprofessional conduct. In 2010, Dr. Nelken was found to have violated a college guideline: "His rental arrangements with MindCare constituted a conflict of interest and were ethically inappropriate" (CPSBC 2010a). The details of his rental agreement and practice administration were classified as a violation with respect to the college-endorsed document "Professional Standards and Guidelines: Conflict of Interest." This document states: "Leasing space to or from third parties in the circumstances identified above if, in exchange, the rental arrangement is markedly different from fair market value and/or the lease arrangements are dependent on the volume of business generated by the physician or third party" (CPSBC 2010b, 2). In another case, Dr. Brown was found to have committed an act of unprofessional conduct: "[He] prescribed clinically excessive quantities of narcotics to his then common-law spouse, and prescribed clinically excessive quantities of stimulants to her then minor son" (CPSBC 2015, 1). Under the college guidelines titled "Professional Standards and Guidelines: Treating Self, Family Members and Those with Whom You Have a Non-professional Relationship," we read: "Physicians must not prescribe narcotic or psychoactive medications to themselves or family members" (CPSBC 2013, 2). These two cases exemplify how a course of action was assessed in relation to the guidelines.

The CPSA also endorses CPGs. This statement appears in the preamble (at the top of page one) for all recommended guidelines (CPSA 2014, 44): "The Standards of Practice of the College of Physicians & Surgeons of Alberta ('the College') are the minimum standards of professional behavior and ethical conduct expected of all regulated members registered in Alberta. Standards of Practice are enforceable under the *Health Professions Act* and will be referenced in the management of complaints and in discipline hearings." There were no cases, however, in which I could find evidence of guidelines being used to discipline the CPSA's members.

There are also cases in which a provincial college does not have a published statement about CPGs. This is true of the CPSNL college orientation guide, for example; however, it does include a statement about resources for doctors to use in their practices, and CPGs are included in the pain management section (CPSNL 2010, 33–38). As another example, the CPSS has a repository of endorsed CPGs, and it states that physicians are recommended to follow them but are also to use "good judgment." There were no exemplary cases of disciplinary actions, however, that provided direct evidence that the guidelines have played a role in any of the CPSS disciplinary adjudications. This could be due to the fact that the nature of the complaints in my sample do not have anything to do with the topics covered in the endorsed guidelines. Then there is the CPSNS (2014), which makes no statement about physicians' use of guidelines in their practices; however, a 2014 decision about Dr. Locke adjudicated improper prescribing practices in accordance with a college-endorsed guideline. The Locke disciplinary statement read:

> However, the auditor concluded that in the management of chronic pain, Dr. Locke *was not practicing within guidelines*. There was no documentation of pain assessments, including the nature and intensity of pain, or the effects of pain on physical and psychological function. No written treatment plans or outcomes to measure success were documented, and there was no documentation of any measure assessing addition risk. (CPSNS 2015, 2, emphasis added)

The decision went on to state that "the auditor concluded that since the previous audit Dr. Locke had made no substantive change in his approach to the prescription of opioids for chronic non-cancer pain and *remained outside the guidelines* and any measure of generally acceptable practice in this area" (CPSNS 2015, 2, emphasis added). So while CPSNS does not state that physicians ought to use college-endorsed guidelines, it openly states that they use them to assess physician misconduct in disciplinary decision statements. The guideline to which the Locke decision refers was also used one year previously in another case: "Dr. Davis does not implement monitoring strategies such as continued reassessment, short dispensing intervals and/or smaller quantities in situations involving potential abuse/misuse or diversion, PMP monitored contracts, urine drug screening, or active use of PMP eAccess for patient profile review" (CPSNS 2014, 3). The infraction was then justified as being misconduct under the following section of the disciplinary decision: "This practice is contrary to the College's Guidelines For The Use of Controlled Substances in the Treatment of Pain; and the Canadian Guideline for Safe and Effective

Use of Opioids for Chronic Non-Cancer Pain" (4). I now turn to a discussion of other instances in which this guideline has been used to determine professional misconduct and as the basis to justify disciplinary action.

Regulating Judgments about Regulated Substances

The most noticeable instances in which college guidelines were used to assess the degree to which a physician's judgment was incorrect had to do with controlled substances – particularly with opioid- and methadone-prescribing practices. These guidelines set the parameters for physician judgments with regard to narcotic prescriptions. I now discuss these cases in detail and compare them to two guidelines that are endorsed by colleges across Canada.

In the next four examples from CPSO, the National Opioid Use Guideline Group's (NOUGG) "Canadian Guideline for Opioids for Chronic Non-Cancer Pain," written in 2010, was used to assess physician conduct. In all four cases, the Discipline Committee's decision regarding unprofessional conduct was determined in relation to the incorrect following of the guideline. NOUGG developed this guideline in response to a "growing need for guidance regarding opioid use for chronic non-cancer pain." Like the sleep medicine document, the opioids document states that the guideline "is intended to educate/inform clinicians and to assist and guide practice decisions ... it is not intended for use as a standard of practice" (NOUGG 2010, 4). While the creators of the guideline may not have intended it to constrain physician judgment, the college's disciplinary decisions are exerting a regulatory effect on clinical judgment.

In the first case, Dr. Van Dorsser (CPSO 2012) was found to have failed to have appropriately managed chronic non-malignant pain. CPSO has endorsed "Evidence-Based Recommendations for Medical Management of Chronic Non-Malignant Pain," which was published in 2000 and is now under review. Dr. Van Dorsser's conduct was deemed unprofessional because he was "prescribing large doses and quantities of narcotics to Patient C, who was known to have a substance abuse disorder and to be at significant risk of overdose because of co-morbidities; and prescribing narcotic medication to Patient D even though he was known to have a substance abuse disorder." According to the first recommendation [R01], the NOUGG (2010) guideline states that physicians ought to conduct a "current, past, and family history of substance use, abuse, and addiction (alcohol, marijuana, tobacco, benzodiazepines, opioids, cocaine, amphetamines, barbiturates, hallucinogens, and solvents)" in order to screen for potentially problematic outcomes (R01). Van Dorsser's judgment was unprofessional because, had he followed the guideline's recommendations to perform a detailed history, he *should have known* about the patient's risk of abusive behaviour.

In the second case, Dr. Reid was found to have "committed an act of professional misconduct, in that he ha[d] failed to maintain the standard of practice of the profession with respect to Patient A, and he ha[d] engaged in disgraceful, dishonourable or unprofessional conduct" (CPSO 2014b). CPSO determined that Reid was culpable of unsafe prescribing practices for opioids. The committee found that Reid had failed to "seek to arrange with a local pharmacy to prescribe opioids to Patient A on the condition that they be dispensed to him in daily or weekly allotments, to reduce the risk of large amounts of medication being lost should events such as theft occur" (ibid.). The guideline makes the following recommendation to lower the risks associated with opioid dependence: physicians should "instruct the pharmacist to dispense daily, twice weekly, or weekly depending on dose and patient reliability" (NOUGG 2010, 72). Second, the committee also found that Reid failed to "require Patient A to undergo regular urine drug screens and pill counts to ensure that he was not overusing or selling the medications" (CPSO 2014b). The guideline recommends that physicians "use urine drug screening to assess compliance" (NOUGG 2010, 86). Third, the committee found that Reid failed to "require Patient A to enter into an opioid agreement that explicitly stated that no early releases or replacement of medications for lost or stolen medications or patches that had fallen off prematurely would be permitted" (CPSO 2014b). The guideline stipulates that early prescription refills are not recommended (NOUGG 2010, 59). Each of these decisions demonstrates that there is evidence to support that CPGs are being used to determine the physician's professional conduct.

Third, Dr. Haines (CPSO 2014a) was found to have failed "to maintain the standard of practice of the profession." First, "there were ongoing prescriptions for opiates and benzodiazepines in patients with substance abuse problems." The NOUGG (2010) guideline states: "Before initiating opioid therapy, ensure comprehensive documentation of the patient's pain condition, general medical condition and psychosocial history, psychiatric status, and substance use history" (R01). Second, Haines was found to have been unprofessional in "combining high dose opiates and benzodiazepines. This combination is known to be a factor in opiate related deaths." The guideline clearly states that "there is evidence that benzodiazepines increase opioid toxicity and risk of overdose" (R06) (NOUGG 2010). The decision also notes that Haines was guilty of "prescribing multiple opiates and multiple benzodiazepines simultaneously. This increases the risk of adverse effects without potential benefit." Further: "Most opioid overdoses involve multiple drugs in addition to opioids" (R06) (NOUGG 2010). The physician ought to have known this and ought to have consulted the guideline for correct prescribing procedures. Finally, the decision found that "two patients were given ongoing prescriptions for opiates without any office assessment for over a year." According to the guideline: "For patients receiving opioids for a prolonged period who may not have had an appropriate trial of therapy, take steps to ensure that long-term therapy is warranted and dose is optimal," including regular urine testing for monitor drug related behaviours (R15) (NOUGG 2010). This last point is similar to the case of Dr. Reid insofar as the physician's judgment failed to ensure patient compliance by using the recommended courses of action and diagnostic tests.

The fourth case of unprofessional conduct that was determined with regard to the incorrect use of the NOUGG guideline is the case of Dr. Nicol (CPSO 2015b). According to the decision: "Dr. Nicol failed to maintain the standard of practice of a general practitioner: in the manner in which he prescribed narcotics to Patient A; in dealing with her underlying substance abuse problem and mood disorder." The decision also makes reference to repeated unprofessional conduct with multiple patients:

> With respect to pain management, he started patients on high-doses of narcotics and, in some cases, mixed varieties, without employing a slower, more cautious approach to the initiation of therapy. Initial screening steps and a clearer recording of functional abilities was lacking. He did not consider drug interactions in his prescribing of medications.

Just as with the case of Dr. Reid, R01 requires a detailed patient history to assess risk (NOUGG 2010). The decision also found that "he was not diligent in minimizing the use of benzodiazepines," which the guideline clearly states in R06 entails a risk of mixing opioid prescriptions (NOUGG 2010). This unprofessional conduct was also found in the case of Dr. Haines.

In Manitoba, the CPSM makes no public statement pertaining to the role of guidelines in disciplinary decisions about professional conduct, but it does list a number of college-endorsed guidelines on its website. The college uses bylaws that regulate the prescription of narcotics (Bylaw #11 Standards of Practice [CPSM 2015]). In 2010, Dr. Hlynka was found to have "issued prescriptions for Percocet or Oxycontin to four categories of people," including "people whom he had never met, or whom he had met, but had not assessed or examined to determine the medical necessity for the narcotics" and "patients for whom he would write prescriptions with no medical rationale, or an inadequate medical rationale" (CPSM 2010, 2). This contravened the college bylaw that required physicians to make assessments about narcotic prescriptions after an examination. Similarly, in 2013 Dr. Coyle was found to have "inappropriately prescribed medications for not less than 10 patients, including narcotics and benzodiazepines and/or opioids, thereby committing acts of professional misconduct" (CPSM 2013). Furthermore, "in many cases, Coyle prescribed medications without any medical justification whatsoever, and without making any entry on the patient's chart" (10). It might be interesting to see if the NOUGG guideline is adopted and later referred to in disciplinary decisions.

Although not explicitly stated in any decision, the NOUGG guideline is playing a role in the Discipline Committee's decision making for adjudicating unprofessional conduct. Prior to turning to a discussion of the effects of this regulatory mechanism, I now discuss a few instances in which the Methadone Management Treatment Program Guideline was used to determine the unprofessional conduct of Dr. Varenbut (CPSO 2015c). In 1999, the CPSO, working in collaboration with the Canadian Centre for Addiction and Mental Health, created a methadone committee. CPSO's role was to represent public interests, educate physicians on addictions medicine, establish guidelines and standards for use of and prescription of methadone, review current practices, and determine who can and who cannot prescribe opioids. The research advisory group for the guideline was to "select and appraise the relevant literature and synthesize the evidence to assist the Guideline authors" (CPSO 2011, 15). The guideline advisory committee defined standards of practice and best practice guidelines, making distinctions between these two concepts (14): standards are principles of patient measurement, based on evidence (synthesized literature), whereas guidelines are recommendations that "assist the MMT physician in *making clinical decisions* about patient care" (16, emphasis added). The guidelines are evidence-based but are not intended to "establish inflexible protocols for patient care nor are they meant to replace the professional judgment of physicians" (16). Again, there is indication that guideline creators do not intend guidelines to constrain expertise or individual judgments.

This guideline, however, was used to assess Dr. Varenbut's conduct. In this case, the decision actually states that the guideline played a role in assessing his conduct: "In 2008, an assessment of Dr. Varenbut's MMT practice based on a review of his care of 15 patients was conducted for the College's Methadone Committee [*sic*]. The Committee concluded that his care of these patients *complied with the MMT Guidelines*" (CPSO 2015c, emphasis added). In the CPSO's 2013 decision, the Discipline Committee made three findings associated with Varenbut's failure to maintain standards of practice:

(a) failing to provide Patient A with a physician appointment within a reasonable time after she sought to be re-admitted to the MMT program in August 2008;

(b) failing to make a timely decision about whether or not to accept Patient A back into the MMT program; and

(c) unreasonably delaying Patient A's access to methadone treatment, of which she was in urgent need. (CPSO 2013c)

Correspondingly, the guideline states: "The MMT physician should conduct a focused physical examination prior to initiating MMT or within a *reasonable* amount of time" (CPSO 2011, 32, emphasis in original). The language of the guideline is similar to that of the decision. The guideline further states: "A patient may be appropriate for initiation on methadone ... if the following circumstances are met ... the patient has been on previous MMT" (33). With respect to finding (c) in Varenbut's case, the physician's conduct was found to be unprofessional insofar as immediate initiation of treatment would have been within the guideline's purview. While, due to privacy laws, there is no public access to patient records, this last decision appears to apply the guideline's recommendations for initiation in light of the physician's familiarity with the patient's history. It relies on the physician's judgment about the patient. The disciplinary decision uses the guideline to illuminate the differences between what happened with the patient (e.g., delay in beginning treatment) with the ideal situation, which is laid out in the normalized expectations of what physicians ought to do with MMT patients.

It is noteworthy that, if the conduct under question has to do with controlled substances like opioids and methadone management, guidelines are predominantly used as a technology of normalization. Contextually, just prior to the Summit and the time range around which my sample was collected, there was a lot of controversy surrounding the dangers and harmful effects of poor opioid prescription management (e.g., Hurwitz 2005; Katz et al. 2011). It is also likely that concerns about the use and prescription of methadone management, which is used to deal with the moral responsibilization of people who struggle with addiction and who ought to stop using illicit drugs – are shaped by both legal and moral concerns. The work of Emma Whelan and Paul Asbridge is helpful with regard to understanding the impetus for regulating these substances. They argue that the push for regulation of these substances came from within medicine, where individual physicians' prescribing practices were problematized: "The attribution of responsibility most often took the form of charges of overzealous or careless prescribing and inadequate follow-up and screening for addiction" (Whelan and Asbridge 2013, 06). Guidelines are meant to be technologies by which physicians can reduce the risk of poor decision making. They are also used to delimit good conduct by legitimizing the differences between poor practices and decision making based on the best available evidence. The use of guidelines to discipline individual practitioners' opioid prescribing practices can be understood as an instance in which the physician's responsibility to know and to act is evaluated in light of the norm, which is spelled out in the appropriate guideline. Given the risk of harm associated with opioid prescriptions and the problematization of both pain and individual physicians' judgments, it is not entirely unsurprising that this area of discipline has received the most attention.[5]

I conclude this section with two more general considerations. The first is a result of the collaborations between the colleges and guideline creators. The NOUGG guideline was endorsed by and created by the CPSO through a partnership between various task forces and groups. Its authors clearly state that guidelines are not intended to replace individual expertise or the astute judgment of the clinician – they aren't meant to constrain the physician or provide "cookbook medicine." Knaapen (2014, 829, emphasis in original), for example, raises the concern that CPGs could "undermine the professional's privileged authority to *evaluate* their own work, as third parties can use guidelines as norms to evaluate the professionals' behaviour." The emerging trend confirms that CPGs are playing a role in normalizing clinical judgments when disciplinary committees need to evaluate what is professional conduct and what is unprofessional conduct. So the evaluation is securing the authority of medicine to evaluate itself. The line between good conduct and misconduct is distributed in relation to the guideline, whether unwittingly or wittingly.[6] Although standards or guidelines are conceived as loose guides to aid decision making, they illuminate the differences between the norm and the actual (i.e., the guideline and the complaint made by the patient, respectively). My data lead me to further explore these normalized judgments as a target of regulatory powers and disciplinary techniques. It is only after the complaints process is initiated that the conduct is assessed, is deemed good or bad, and disciplinary powers are deployed. If guidelines are meant as decision-making aids, not as a replacement for clinical judgment, but are being used to normalize and draw the line between good conduct and bad conduct, then what exactly is their goal? Getting physicians to know the evidence, on the one hand, while simultaneously producing the effect of rule-following (lest they be subject to disciplinary action) on the other? Getting them to make decisions in line with the guidelines rather than assessing the evidence and evaluating the recommendation?

Sociological work has examined how guidelines are a result of a changing professional landscape. Waring (2007, 164) argues that "the future of medical regulation and also medical/managerial relations may not be characterized by expanding the domains of management over medicine, but rather expanding the domains of management within medicine." His research explores how doctors used guidelines to justify their decisions across several departments of a United Kingdom hospital. Using guidelines allowed physicians to avoid having someone else scrutinize their decisions. Waring's take on this phenomenon is that guidelines are but another response to the questioning of medical authority from within medicine: "In being adaptive and seeking to limit managerial involvement, doctors are seemingly re-articulating what it means to self-regulate, absorbing managerial assumptions and recreating themselves as the managers" (176). While Waring shows how guidelines can be used to resist legislative encroachments on the profession, I now explain how they rely on emergent conceptualization of clinical judgment.

The Professional Regulation of What?

Mitchell Dean (1994, 196) explicates the link between discipline and modes of subjectification: "The genealogy of punitive practices in *Discipline and Punish* invoked four dimensions in order to make intelligible the transformation of the forms of punishment: the punishable substance, the mode of subjectification of the punished, the punitive work or self-forming activity, and the telos or mode of being in which the penalty is incorporated." With regard to evidence-based guidelines, the disciplinary substance is the judgment, the mode of subjectification is found in CPGs, the punitive work is located in the sanction (such as having to complete continuing medical education), and the objective is to use evidence to improve medical care. Here I explain how the discursive practice of clinical judgment is successfully regulated through the normalizing judgments of disciplinary decisions. These disciplinary decisions embody unarticulated assumptions about clinical judgment. The use of guidelines as a solution to the problematization of clinical judgment presupposes that it is possible to identify good and bad judgments and to punish those judgments that are incorrect. My analysis of disciplinary decisions reveals the ontological assumptions that lie behind clinical judgment and that underpin the disciplinary structure.

To explain the nature of these assumptions, I describe Foucault's project and compare it to my findings to justify my claims about the ontology of clinical judgments. In making this comparison, I explain *what* is regulated and normalized by disciplinary actions. I shift my analysis away from the human subject and focus on the relations that structure the disciplinary substance. In *The Use of Pleasure,* Michel Foucault (1985, 24) sets out to study the problematization of sexual practice. He approaches this genealogical work with a study of moral statements about the use and regulation of pleasures from antiquity to early Christianity. He defines morality as "a set of values and rules of action that are recommended to individuals through the intermediary of various prescriptive agencies" (25). Values and rules are codified in explicit doctrines. A CPG is a moral code: it recommends to individual doctors how they ought to act in their medical practices. Rules and values are transmitted in a diffuse manner, comprising "a complex interplay of elements that counterbalance and correct one another, and cancel each other out on certain points, thus providing for compromises or loopholes" (ibid.). Diffuse forms of morality in medicine, however, are found in the "hidden curriculum" (cf. Haas and Shaffir 1982) of medical education. For example, the horizontal program at McMaster comprises professional conventions about attitudes and interactions with other medical staff, departments, practitioners, and/or one's bedside manner.

Foucault specifies that morality also "refers to the real behavior of individuals in relation to the rules and values that are recommended to them." The difference between the rule and the conduct is measured by making a normalizing judgment: morality "thus designates the manner in which they comply more or less fully with a standard of conduct, the manner in which they obey or resist an interdiction or a prescription; the manner in which they respect or disregard a set of values" (Foucault 1985, 25). Codes of conduct stipulate the correct or good course of action for the ethical subject. Those physicians who use guidelines to "assist" with their decision making are following the manner in which the colleges are making judgments about conduct (NOUGG 2010). As discussed, EBM also prescribes how physicians ought to conduct themselves: by "conducting a detailed appraisal of the methods and results" of medical studies before making their decisions (Fowkes and Fulton 1991, 1140).

Codes of conduct have a normative authority that prescribes the manner in which subjects ought to act with regard to themselves so as to become good members of groups, institutions, or society more generally. The ethical subject is defined with reference to "the manner in which one ought to form oneself as an ethical subject acting in reference to the prescriptive elements that make up the code." Analytically, the substance of the ethical subject is determined in relation to the degrees of difference between the rule and the subject's conduct, which means that there are "different ways for the acting individual to operate, not just as an agent, but as an ethical subject of this action" (Foucault 1985, 26). Foucault uses conjugal fidelity between marital partners as an example of a moral code that prescribes what constitutes good conduct: being faithful. There are many ways to practise fidelity, which provides a number of ethical choices for subjects to make. These choices comprise four analytical points.

The first concerns the "determination of the ethical substance," which is defined as "the ways in which the individual has to constitute this or that part of himself as the prime material of his moral conduct" (Foucault 1985, 26). In Foucault's example, fidelity concerns prohibitions on one's actions: sleeping with someone who is not your spouse is prohibited. But fidelity can also require resisting the desire one might develop for another partner. The prime material of the ethical substance is more than just carrying out the act of only sleeping with one's spouse: the ethical substance is the relationship between oneself and one's desires. In the case of medicine, CPGs lay out a course of action, which is a code used by disciplinary committees to determine the shades of difference between professional- and non-professional conduct. The substance of disciplinary decisions is the judgment that "failed to maintain the standards of the profession." The committee constitutes the material of moral conduct through normalizing judgment: each judgment is assessed by the committee as potentially inferior, not up to date, relying on conventionalisms or subjective opinions or intuitions. Under the code, the physician ought to uphold the standards of the profession and use the best evidence. Maintaining the standards of the profession relies on the assumption that good conduct is consistent with guidelines because the latter are evidence-based and stipulate recommended actions. The sanction for not following guidelines reveals that what physicians ought to act on is their use of evidence, which relies on deferring their own judgments to a code, a guideline that has remedied the shortcomings of their ability to judge.

Foucault's second analytical point concerns the various modes of subjection, which are defined as "the way in which the individual establishes his relation to the rule and recognizes himself as obliged to put it into practice." Under the moral code of fidelity, one's subjective relationship to being faithful can be through personal religious belief – for example, one ascribes to the religious practices associated with conjugal fidelity and adheres to them. There is also the notion that one has a duty, a responsibility to revive or maintain that spiritual belief or tradition (Foucault 1985, 27). In EBM, the code rests on the assumption that the physician is committed to self-learning, to keeping up with the best evidence. And, given the social circumstances (e.g., time constraints, too much information), this means reading and familiarizing oneself with CPGs and best practice statements. There is an assumption that if physicians are reading guidelines, they will follow the recommendations because they are based on the best available evidence. The college disciplinary decisions also indicate that there is an obligation for the physician to establish her judgment in relation to the CPGs, knowing when to follow them and uphold them for the good of the profession.

Foucault refers to the "ethical work," sometimes called the "elaboration of the self," as the third analytical point. This is the work "that one performs on oneself, not only in order to bring one's conduct into compliance with a given rule, but to attempt to transform oneself into the ethical subject of one's behavior" (Foucault 1985, 27). This form of work, Foucault says, is lifelong insofar as it requires that, for example, the subject commits his life to sexual austerity. Even violations are opportunities to learn and reevaluate one's relationship to the rule. I think about this in terms of Alcoholics Anonymous (AA) as well, where abstinence is the renunciation of alcohol, which requires both practising the steps and making the setbacks meaningful. Should one "fall off the wagon," the AA member has an opportunity to devote himself to understanding the twelve steps, which is part of "the process." In the disciplinary cases I reviewed, the sanctions against the physicians often included a requirement to enrol in continued medical education courses. For example, in the case of Dr. Reid, the CPSO (2014b) ordered that he both: "participate in and successfully complete the Safe Opioid Prescribing program offered by the University of Toronto, or an equivalent program acceptable to the College" and "participate in and successfully complete the Understanding Boundaries in Managing the Risks Inherent in the Doctor-Patient Relationship course offered by Western University, or an equivalent program acceptable to the College." The education provides opportunities for retraining, for Dr. Reid to recognize his violation of the rule as well as the CPGs on best practice and to measure his conduct in relation to his ability to recover and improve from this experience. The disciplinary decision rests on the assumption that physicians can do ethical work to bring their future conduct into accordance with the moral rules. Should physicians wish to keep their licence and to keep practising medicine, they must freely enrol in these courses and improve their conduct.

The fourth and final analytical point highlights the objective of ethical work, what Foucault called the "telos" of the ethical subject:

> An action is not only moral in itself, in its singularity; it is also moral in its circumstantial integration and by virtue of the place it occupies in a pattern of conduct ... A moral act tends toward its own accomplishment; it also aims beyond [it] ... to the establishing of a moral conduct that commits an individual, not only to other actions always in conformity with values and rules, but to a certain mode of being, a mode of being characteristic of the ethical subject. (Foucault 1985, 27–28)

For example, practising fidelity has different "goals," such as the salvation of the soul or mastery over one's desires. For the act to count as moral, it must be committed in relation to the value of the rule as an end in itself and not be reducible to a series of acts that just conforms to the rule (Foucault 1985, 28). The value of using CPGs is that generalized rules based on evidence are good in and of themselves. To fail to apply these rules to particular cases, as I observed in disciplinary decisions, was to question the value of evidence within the medical profession. One of the goals of guidelines implementation is to improve health care (e.g., CMA 2007, 2011). The use of CPGs demonstrates that it is the duty of individual clinicians to act so as to attain that goal by following the recommendations within CPGs. This is indicated by the statements within the guidelines. Their purpose is not to replace clinical judgment but, rather, to function as technologies to aid in decision making. The disciplinary committees, however, evaluate how judgments integrated CPGs into the clinical circumstances. This demonstrates that subjects ought to recognize their duty to improve health care by acting according to evidence-based guidelines. The value of the use of evidence – as the technique by which to improve health care – supersedes the series of acts required to assess and appraise the evidence.

Following Foucault's line of reasoning on the ethical substance of codes, which are used to discipline and normalize individual conduct in the clinic, I do not look for a history of behaviours that would measure the extent to which the actions of individuals were actually consistent with the rules; instead, in a genealogical analysis of the emergence of clinical epidemiology, I indicate its links to EBM, its justification for institutionalized education reform, and its targeting of the thoughts and action (clinical judgments) of physicians. In so doing I show that it is the technologies of EBM that are understood as forms of moral subjectivation – the practices, to paraphrase Foucault (1985, 29), that are meant to ensure the amelioration of clinical judgment with the use of evidence. For Foucault, and for my research, codes of behaviour and modes of subjectivation are intertwined. Where there are moral codes, there are authorities that enforce them and require that duties are learned and observed – or sanctioned when they are not: "The subjectivation[7] occurs ... where the ethical subject refers his conduct to a law, to which he must submit at the risk of committing offense that may make him liable to punishment" (29–30). The relations of power enact sanctions for the failure to follow the rule, which influences the ethical subject's decision to comply.

While disciplinary action may provoke the idea that physicians are incentivized to use CPGs and deterred from acting without or against them, that is not the complete story. Each provincial medical act endows the colleges with the authority to regulate their members, and any contravention of the act risks a disciplinary hearing and the offending member is liable to sanctions imposed by the college. Consider the CPSO, where acts of professional misconduct concern "an act or omission relevant to the practice of medicine that, having regard to all the circumstances, would reasonably be regarded by members as disgraceful, dishonourable or unprofessional" (Section 33, Medicine Act, 1991, Ontario). It is the responsibility of the individual member to act reasonably, which means, given measures of best practice, being a lifelong learner, keeping up with new information, and acting on the best evidence. The disciplinary committee only deals with those cases that are brought under its authority. By normalizing and sanctioning on the basis of guidelines, the committee assumes that physicians ought to practise EBM, and the appropriate courses of action are spelled out in the guidelines it uses to measure the conduct of individual cases. Those judgments that are unprofessional are also "immoral" (disgraceful) in light of the CPGs used to measure conduct.

Which brings our analysis back to the horizontal program at McMaster, which sought to instill an attitude in the physician that would ensure that she was self-motivated and staying abreast of the best information as a value in and of itself. The individualized ethical subject is not only about passive rule-following but also about attitude: "More important than the content of the law and its conditions of application was the attitude that caused one to respect it [the code]" (Foucault 1985, 31). Programs of conduct that prescribe actions also prescribe ways of being, individual orientations to those actions, where the value of doing it is over and above the acts that comprise it. For Foucault's project, the Greek practice of sophrosyne, whereby individuals are educated about desires, is about one's attitude towards the value of knowing oneself as an object of knowledge, an attitude towards the value of measuring and thinking about and rationalizing one's desires (62). It is an ontological question about the nature of knowing the self, how one ought to be in relation to the code, not only what one must do. In the case of CPGs, disciplinary decisions assume that physicians must recognize not only the possible sanctions for acting against recommendations but also the value of acting on evidence – that health care will get better if everyone does their part, that improved health care is intrinsically valuable. The physician ought to recognize that the assessment of the evidence has been performed in advance by others, and so her critical appraisal is not necessary. The ethical substance of judgments is an externalized judgment, one understood to defer to the authority of the guidelines, their objectives, and the disciplinary committee that uses them to punish. The mode of subjectivation requires that physicians be deresponsibilized in relation to the code, that they recognize that they ought not to judge but to follow the guidelines. The mechanism that deresponsibilizes their judgment in relation to the code is the normalizing judgment of the disciplinary committees.

5

The Impossible Clinic: Biopolitics, Governmentality, and Liberalism

THIS CHAPTER SPELLS out my contribution to the sociology of evidence-based medicine. I argue that EBM is an impossible project: it is set up in such a way that it cannot achieve its own aims. To make this claim, I draw on Foucault's concept of dispositif to show how the strategies of EBM perpetuate existing hierarchies. By looking at research in biopower and biopolitics in the sociology of health and medicine, I explain why EBM is able to continue, despite the fact that responsibilized judgments may not be achieved. Finally, I show that, although liberal forms of government rely on self-governance strategies, professional disciplinary strategies that normalize using codes of conduct in order to regulate have the potential to deresponsibilize those who depend on them. This encourages governmentality studies to consider that not all liberal governance strategies enlist individuals in self-development, that some strategies constitute professional subjects who externalize judgment by relying on codes of conduct.

The professional colleges use CPGs to discipline, and this fact presents an opportunity to understand the role of these technologies of power in normalizing medical practice through tribunal judgments. EBM, and clinical epidemiology before that, sought to resolve the problems of clinical practice by bridging the gap between science and practice to pacify public concerns over medical authority (and from within the profession as well). The critical appraisal method was taught in medical programs so that students would become self-learners and, throughout their careers, would evaluate and "critically appraise" the evidence for themselves, both keeping up with new information and avoiding the pitfalls of conventionalism. The use of guidelines to measure whether a judgment was good or bad shifts the responsibility away from the physician's ability to appraise the evidence and towards the capacity of the physician to know a rule and follow it. This would seem to support Greenhalgh and colleagues' (2014) concern that EBM is increasing the emphasis on rule-following in the clinic.

But why has this failure of EBM stabilized in the regulatory technologies of professional medicine? To answer this question, I turn to the final element in Foucault's analysis of social apparatuses and their formation. The final element necessary to establish the existence of a dispositif is, to paraphrase Foucault, to be able to understand the place of the strategy in relation to the play of dominations, power relations, and struggles (Foucault 1980a).[1] The effects of the contingent conjuncture of the relations of EBM discourse and the strategies of education and regulation are both responsibilizing and deresponsibilizing. The responsible clinician with good judgment uses CPGs, but the normalization of professional judgment produces the opposite effect, which is, in fact, counter-productive to EBM's strategy to optimize clinical judgment via the surveillance of the implementation of evidence in any given physician's practice. This is a failure of EBM because the mechanisms that deploy its knowledge with the objective of overseeing and necessitating the use of evidence undermines the possibility of its achieving its goals.

The criterion for being able to claim that EBM has become a social apparatus is evident when the sociologist can isolate the usage of these effects and explain how they perpetuate existing hierarchies. Foucault details the importance of this criterion in *Discipline and Punish* when he explains that the effects of the penitentiary technique for punishing delinquents actually indicate the failure of the prison. If the goals of the prison are to punish humanely, to correct delinquents by educating them, and to reduce crime and offences (cf. Foucault 1979, 270–71), the prison fails. He goes on: "If the prison-institution has survived for so long, with such immobility, if the principle of penal detention has never seriously been questioned, it is no doubt because this carceral system was deeply rooted and carried out certain very precise functions" (271). The "function" of these failures is the facilitation of broader advantages to dominant groups. In the words of Alan Hunt (2004, 606), genealogical analysis must distinguish "the mechanisms through which ... discourses work" and also show how these mechanisms "can work to favour some and to disadvantage others." In *Discipline and Punish*, Foucault explains how the delinquent enters into forms of supervision within the prison and then beyond (e.g., the police record), which enables the administration and exploitation of illegalities: "Arms trafficking ... or more recently drug trafficking show a similar functioning of this 'useful delinquency': the existence of a legal prohibition creates around it a field of illegal practices, which one manages to supervise, while extracting from it an illicit profit through elements, themselves illegal, but rendered manipulable by their organization in delinquency" (Foucault 1979, 280). These kinds of setups perpetuate existing class hierarchies as those who leave prison have a hard time finding employment (300) and so return to a life of (for example), drug dealing: ex-cons sell drugs to the upper class. It benefits the upper class to have delinquents who can secure the trafficking of drugs to replenish their supply. It is not, however, the upper class that "uses" the prison to produce the drug dealers it needs. Foucault concludes that power relations reproduce these relations of domination and perpetuate the existence of the prison. The goal of Foucault's analytic is to articulate the relations of force that perpetuate institutional failures and, in so doing, benefit other forms of domination.

What is served by the failure of EBM? In order to answer this question, I discuss the convergence of the disciplinary and normalizing powers of biopower and biopolitics as well as the governance strategies of advanced liberalism. I argue that the failure of EBM allows liberal forms of governmentality to perpetuate.

Biopower/Biopolitics

The effects of EBM occur within a biopolitical dispositif that allows them to perpetuate. Here I explain the elements of biopower/biopolitics and apply them to justify my argument that EBM continues despite its failures because it exists within a dispositif that perpetuates liberal forms of governance. Examining these elements allows me to shift my focus from biopolitics to liberalism because, as Foucault points out, understanding biopolitics requires understanding the liberal apparatus of governing. I demonstrate that the antithetical effects of EBM signal the failure of liberal objectives of control within institutionalized programs of conduct whose goal is to "secure" freedom.

Volume 1 of Foucault's (1978, 143) *History of Sexuality* uses the term "bio-power to designate what brought life and its mechanisms into the realm of explicit calculations and made knowledge-power an agent of transformation of human life." Foucault's work analyzes the deployment of sexuality as a discourse that makes life a political object by joining together forces that maximize the capacities of the body and the control of a species body, a population. With regard to my research, this form of power intersects with the relations of discourse that produce knowledge about clinical practice: medicine was one institution in which the improvement of the life of the population was assigned to the individual judgment of the physician. Clinical epidemiology was one scientific discourse that brought the clinical management of life into the realm of measurement, where the effectiveness of therapy and medical intervention could provide information about the efficiency of clinical work. This science brought clinical practice into what Foucault calls the "domain of value and utility": "Such a power has to quantify, measure, appraise, and hierarchize ... it effects distributions around the norm" (144). Using biostatistical methods and study designs such as the randomized controlled trial, knowledge about medical interventions could be surveilled, collected, and ranked in accordance with scientific principles of validity. Where EBM takes place is at the level of the individual:

EBM individualizes the responsibility of physicians to appraise and rank the evidence for themselves. Clinical epidemiology provides a method for distributing the knowledge of clinical effectiveness: therapies are measured in relation to population health, and the best therapies appear in best practice recommendations.

For Foucault, "a power whose task it is to take charge of life needs continuous regulatory and corrective mechanisms." In Canadian medicine this task falls to the medical colleges and entails the ability to monitor physicians to ensure that they are lifelong learners, constantly keeping up with the best therapies and new clinical methods to implement in their practices. The role of the college is regulatory insofar as it has the authority to discipline its members and has access to the guidelines that serve to justify the regulation of professional conduct. On Foucault's (1980b, 144) terrain, the use of codes to regulate is normalizing, and "a normalizing society is the historical outcome of a technology of power centred on life." The clinic becomes the setting in which society can intervene and ameliorate health. The target of these strategies for regulating the health of the population becomes the individual encounter between physicians and their patients.

The objective of modern moral and governmental programs is constituted by "a power to *foster* life" and to improve on it, ameliorate it, and encourage its flourishing (Foucault 1978, 138, emphasis in original). The disciplinary actions taken against physicians aim to encourage the flourishing of a healthy society through the trustworthiness of medicine (e.g., CMA 2004). For Foucault, the relations of power that control life are linked between disciplines of the body and regulatory controls. Foucault refers to these two poles as biopower and biopolitics, respectively. Biopower is "an anatomopolitics of the body" and concerns "the body as a machine," specifically through the following operations: "Its disciplining, the optimization of its capabilities, the extortion of its forces, the parallel increase of its usefulness and its docility, its integration into systems of efficient and economic controls" (139). My research shows that individualizing technologies such as CPGs discipline the capacities of the physician's judgment in the clinic. CPGs are underpinned by the assumption that the clinician's judgment can be ameliorated by best practice rules, and the colleges are the mechanisms that ensure its regulation. Further, CPGs target the capacity of the physician's judgment and aim to optimize it through normalizing codes, and they subjectivize clinical subjects that ought not to judge evidence but, rather, execute best practice. In other words, CPGs harness the capabilities of judgment and externalize it.

The use of CPGs in the clinic are justified in the name of regulatory control over the health care system. The Health Council of Canada was created in order to improve health care and to equalize the health care system across all provinces. Foucault would view these sorts of initiatives as having a biopolitical objective, where the concern is with "propagation and longevity, with all the conditions that can cause these to vary" (Foucault 1978, 139). Biopolitical interventions depend on regulatory controls. Although the HCC began as a reporting mechanism, as a system of surveilling discrepancies in health care systems across the country, its eventual intervention into population health came to target the individual clinical encounter. EBM was deployed as a solution to the problems associated with the clinic as it provided a scientific rationale and method for remedying problematized clinical judgment. Best practice, the HCC and CMA reasoned, required the improvement of individual judgment rather than, for example, the improvement of health infrastructure[2] – a systematic assessment of medical resources was not the dominant problematization within the field of medicine. Colleges disciplined on an individual basis rather than on the evaluation of the clinical environment or system.

Foucault argues that the emergence of biopolitics was intertwined with liberal forms of rule. Liberalism belongs to a terrain of political discourse that "constitutes ... criticism of previous governmentality that one is trying to get free" (Foucault 2008, 320). EBM belongs to a criticism of previous forms of medical authority and practice: it seeks to correct the abuses of subjective judgments, conventional wisdom, and the reliance on intuition rather than evidence. Because liberalism is also premised on the importance of individual freedoms, corrective measures for the "old regime" of "doctor knows best" tended to focus on individual choices. To recall the words of Eddy (1990a), the solution to the problematized aspects of clinical care and the threats to clinical authority lay in improving the capacity of doctors to make good decisions, and CPGs were one such solution.

But the freedom to make better choices is another problematic aspect of liberal rule. Foucault explains that fundamental to liberalism is a tension between freedom and security. Freedom is considered an essential, natural right within liberal forms of rule (Foucault 2008, 63). But within these relations of discourse freedom is problematic as it must be assessed on the basis of enabling and constraining freedom of choice: "Freedom is never anything other ... than an actual relation between governors and governed, a relation in which the measure of the 'too little' existing freedom is given by the 'even more' freedom demanded" (ibid.). With challenges to medical authority from the public, various social sciences, government, and the field of medicine, it was difficult to determine how to allow the judgment of doctors to flourish. The reform of medical education that began in the relations of discourse and was then later institutionalized at McMaster can be understood as an effort relating to the "management and organization of the conditions in which one can be free" (ibid.). Physicians were encouraged to make better judgments by learning to assess the evidence and continue to learn on their own, which required the medical colleges to provide the guidelines and resources necessary, as well as the requisite controls and incentives, to ensure that physicians were able to keep up. According to Foucault, "liberalism must produce freedom, this very act entails the establishment of limitations, controls, forms of coercion, and obligations relying on threats" (64). To explain this point, Foucault uses the example of free trade: in order to guarantee freedom within the market for actors to buy and sell "freely," there must also exist regulatory mechanisms that control and limit certain actions, such as preventing monopolies (e.g., anti-monopoly legislation), to ensure the freedom for all. Analogously, in medicine, each province has its own medical act, which regulates both the actions of doctors and the rights of the profession to self-govern.

According to Foucault (2008, 65), in liberal forms of rule, the principle of calculation for the cost of maintaining freedom is security: "The problem of security is the protection of collective interest against individual interests ... The freedom of the workers must not become a danger for the enterprise." In the case of medicine, individual judgments came to be problematized in the relations of discourse, and it was determined that "bad" judgments threatened the authority of medicine as an enterprise. In order to ensure that the threats to medical authority would not become ammunition for state-regulated oversight or control over the medical profession, it became imperative to set up a range of disciplinary techniques that delineated the (professional) conduct of individuals (cf. Foucault 2008, 66). Disciplinary techniques, like those Foucault (1979) observes in the birth of the prison, emerged at the same historical moment as liberalism. Biopolitical programs aim to intervene in the health of the population (i.e., health care) and also to problematize the freedom of individuals (i.e., clinical judgments). Thus, the implementation of CPGs as normalizing codes of conduct can be understood within a liberal governmental strategy.

Governmentality Studies and the Sociology of Medicine

I have shown how physicians were deresponsibilized as a consequence of the convergence of professional mechanisms of regulation and the biopolitical objectives of liberal governance strategies. The biopolitical regulation of health through programs that target individual clinical judgments can be further explained by engaging with governmentality studies in the social sciences. I now explain the effects of professional and liberal governance strategies. The medical colleges' normalization of clinical judgment not only governs the clinic "at a distance" but also provides

an occasion for sociology to reconsider its understanding of subjectivity and the ethical dimensions of self-governance.

Foucault (2003, 244) describes governmentality as a product
of the emergence of a specific form of knowledge collected about
society: "The ensemble formed by the institutions, procedures,
analyses, and reflections, the calculations and tactics that allow
the exercise of this very specific albeit complex form of power,
which has as its target population, as its principal form of knowledge political economy, and as its essential technical means apparatuses of security." Modern governance, according to Foucault,
is characterized by a need for an extensive knowledge-production
apparatus about (social) life with the objective of improving it.
Knowledge is collected about target populations. Apparatuses of
security are concerned with securing the conditions under which
the life of the population can be enhanced and developed through
individual choice. As a technology of EBM, CPGs aim to produce
the conditions, in the form of general rules, that would control
for variation in health care delivery. This can be observed in the
words of the HCC, which holds that CPGs have the objective of
improving health care and the "health outcomes of Canadians."
The guidelines govern the possible choices that a doctor can make
or not make in a clinical encounter. Foucault (1982, 221) defines
governing as follows: "To govern is to structure the possible field
of actions of others"; thus, governing is "the conduct of conduct."
By delimiting the possible decisions and courses of action that
a physician may take with a particular patient, CPGs provide a
means through which the range of her possible actions is secured.
For example, the guidelines lay out the correct course of action
for correct opioid prescriptions and monitoring. Not only are the
choices about how to prescribe and who is to prescribe delimited,
there are also detailed instructions (NOUGG 2010) in R06 to surveille and monitor patient populations who are on opioids. The
physicians' choices are structured to govern opioid users through
the institution of medicine.

By "disseminating best practices," the HCC's objective of ameliorating health care by controlling for practice variation emphasizes

intervention at the level of individualized clinical judgment. This is consistent with governmentality studies, which show that governing strategies are often actualized to "manage the habits and activities of subjects to achieve that end" (Rose, O'Malley and Valverde 2006, 84), which reveals a normative dimension to governmental strategies: the courses of possible action that doctors can take are pre-structured on this basis of improving health outcomes. The link between the institution of medicine and governmental objectives is visible in the CPGs meant to resolve problems associated with the individual clinical encounter. EBM's failure is that it allows for the ongoing individualization of responsibility to improve health care, which is a tenet of liberal governance. Liberal strategies channel the effects of EBM (both its responsibilizing and deresponsibilizing effects), individualizing the cost-effectiveness of health care to the clinical encounter, which allows the administration of health care to tout fiscal responsibility while not regulating the freedom of medical practitioners "too much."

Before turning to a discussion of the function of the failure of EBM, I first want to explain the relevance of the effect of deresponsibilization to the field of governmentality studies. In this field, power is operationalized by articulating three levels on which governmental programs operate: economic, social life, and individual conduct (Rose and Miller 1992, 173). Rose's work on governmentality and advanced liberalism, in particular, stresses that governmental programs that individualize in order to improve a population outcome are products of specific liberal forms of governance. The objectives of this form of governance are met, ideally, through the choices of individuals. In the case under study, this would be the physicians following CPGs.

The responsibility to improve population health problematizes a series of choices that the physician must make in the clinic, and the CPGs are implemented to resolve these issues "at a distance" – it is still up to the physician to use the CPGs or not, and "expertise" and clinical judgment are encouraged in the CPGs I examine in Chapter 4. The physician is conceived as an ethical subject, meaning that she or he must make a decision about what is right in the face of clinical uncertainties and potential sanctions should that choice be incorrect. The problematization of choice in liberal governance constitutes an ethical dilemma for the subject: "Choice is difficult for the individual because of the pluralization of expertise about risk, which provides not only different calibrations of uncertainty but also paradoxical and sometimes contradictory recommendations about how to act responsibly." The problematization of clinical judgment is ongoing, as is the proliferation and pluralization of guidelines. The same condition often has conflicting guidelines, depending on which database one consults. As a result, individuals must "become their own policy makers, charting principled courses of action that exhibit their capacity for self-improvement in self-controlled ways" (Erickson and Doyle 2003, 114). Physicians are positioned by the demands to use evidence and CPGs in relation to the need to demonstrate their ethical capacity to make good judgments.

The provincial college endorsement regulates the variation associated with choice. In the regulation of the problematized risks associated with clinical judgment, individuals are "held to the responsible standards established by the institutions concerned, regardless of whether she accepts responsibility on the personal level" (Erickson and Doyle 2003, 114). My examination of disciplinary decisions is evidence that, when a complaint process is initiated, the guidelines act as standards to measure the difference between the ideal decision and the actual outcome. Physicians are disciplined regardless of whether they thought they made a bad judgment or not. The deployment of guidelines for normalizing judgments about clinical decisions produces an obligation on the part of physicians: they must become masters of their judgment, which would mean externalizing it to the guidelines. In the governmentality literature, this ethical duty is referred to a "self-governance" tactic, and it "refers to the significant consequence of responsibilization, namely, the requirement that individuals seek out and fashion an ethical life for themselves." Hunt's work is helpful for understanding how the subject's responsibility is constituted not around the content of the decision but, rather, around the recognition that it is necessary to be responsible to one's obligations. In the case of medical practice, the commitment of the lifelong learner requires physicians to see that their practices are in line with their responsibility for making good judgments. According to Hunt (2003, 172), "this requirement does not impose prescriptions about the correct conduct of that life. It only demands that life be conducted reflexively, or that the individual be capable of advancing some justification of the choices made." EBM requires that judgments be backed up by good evidence. The professional disciplinary decisions are no exception: they delimit the nature of good decisions as externalized to CPGs, which is justified by the latter's being evidence-based. The CPGs recommend specific content, but the clinician is obligated to recognize the necessity of using evidence to make their decisions.

For Foucault (1985, 13), moral codes serve as "functional devices that would enable individuals to question their own conduct, to watch over and give shape to it, and to shape themselves as ethical subjects." Rules for conduct allow individuals to understand their responsibilities and to fashion their life according to those codes. The work of Nikolas Rose expands on this notion of self-development, of the ethical duties that constitute the subject of normalization. Rose's (2007, 27) concept of "ethopolitics" is defined as "the self-techniques by which human beings should judge and act on themselves to make themselves better than they are." Similar to Hunt's point about responsibilization (see above), Rose posits that subjects have an ethical obligation to reflect on their choices and to act in ways that are considered good, in line with the authorities that have specific objectives, whose success depends on the individual choices of the subject. My formulation of medical practice has implications for considering the intersection between 1) the tactics by which individuals shape themselves in light of modes of subjectivation and 2) codes of conduct. On the one hand, the ethical obligations for physicians to reflect on their clinical judgments can be explained by the concept of ethopolitics (as they determine the self-techniques according to which they should act); on the other hand, physicians must not judge – they ought to use guidelines, despite EBM's insistence on critically appraising the evidence. So, according to the politics of ethical self-governance, the act of judging may end up being externalized. The nature of this process is regulated through the professional mechanisms that rely on a deresponsibilized ontology of the modes of subjectivation by which subjects come to self-govern. Understanding the relationship between ethical subjects and their self-governance should be expanded to include the externalizing effects of the normalizing strategies of regulation.

I now turn to the broader social conditions that enable these forms of regulation and, in doing so, show how the failure of EBM benefits liberal biopolitical governance strategies. Thomas Osborne discusses the authority of the profession of medicine with regard to the problem of governing, asking how medicine comes to concern itself with the problems of governing professional conduct. According to Osborne, this question has to do with the construction of truth in the clinic. Drawing on an engagement with Foucault's *The Birth of the Clinic,* Osborne argues that the regulation of truth production was problematized in the clinical hospital but that this process had to be governed "at a distance," whereby "the public must delegate to the state not direct control over medical acts but control over the producer of those acts ... that is, [it must] regulat[e] the 'competence' of the subject of medical truth." The subject of medical truth is the physician who ought to examine the patient's body and make statements about the cause, condition, prognosis, and so on of the patient's problem. It was through the production of seeing and saying that the truth of the body could be produced. It is the liberal commitments of medicine that ground the normalizing judgments about the competence of medical acts. Medical disciplinary hearings make those determinations by looking at the producer of medical truths, the acting subject (the physician), rather than, say, the infrastructure of the health care system. This process requires that individual conduct and competence in the production of truth must be "indexed" in relation to the ideal of the profession (Osborne 1993, 346). EBM is underpinned by liberal questions of governance as medical truths must be produced by relying on evidence, which is produced through the discursive relations of clinical epidemiology. It is the responsibility of the physician to keep up with evidence so that she is able to make truth statements about diagnoses and treatment options and interventions. When complaints are filed, the profession assesses the physician's conduct with an eye to the CPG index, which is formulated according to the ideal use of such evidence. The physician under question assesses the use of evidence pertaining to her individual conduct as a professional regulatory strategy.

In liberal societies, the state gives the medical profession the responsibility to regulate matters of public health. Osborne draws on a historical example from the United Kingdom, where the state charged medical officers across the country with the responsibility for monitoring and controlling the spread of cholera (Osborne 1993, 351). In my research, the liberal aspects of governance can be observed when the HCC gave the Canadian Medical Association the task of creating a database of CPGs. Because the state allows medicine to self-regulate, the monitoring of the use and implementation of CPGs was delegated to the provincial medical colleges. These colleges, to fulfill their regulatory role, would have to assess the competent use of these guidelines. So what kinds of subject positions are constituted in the liberal mandate to self-regulate?

As discussed earlier, liberalism seeks to reconcile individual freedom with the control of the outcomes of individual practices in relation to a particular objective: "Liberalism involves a network of diverse techniques and practices through which the governed are constituted as autonomous subjects and are encouraged to exercise their freedom in appropriate ways" (Fournier 1999, 283). Guidelines in medicine state that it remains the task of the physician to assess and decide what is best for the patient. Fournier's work on governmentality and the professions demonstrates that "professional labour is autonomous labour where the conditions of autonomy have already been inscribed in particular forms of conduct articulated in the notion of 'professional competence'" (282). In medicine, the provincial medical acts detail what kinds of acts are professional and acceptable; the moral force of this is exercised through discipline in the form of both professional hearings and sanctions. The CPGs "inscribe" particular forms of conduct, recommending courses of action for practitioners. These subject positions are devised by experts and stakeholders. The doctors who are supposed to use them are *users* not judgers; at the same time, the CPGs state that they are not meant to replace expertise. The implementation of CPGs maintained the hierarchy of authority among the government, the profession, and the clinic.

Further, liberal rationality inscribes the power to discipline to the provincial colleges, which, in turn, produces what Fournier (1999, 283) refers to as "subject positions and the definition of moral conduct." Liberal governance justifies moral programs of conduct (such as the endorsement of CPGs) to delineate good professional conduct through scientific expertise since doing so "serves to constitute human beings as autonomous subjects with a responsibility ... to conduct their life in appropriate ways" (284). CPGs appeal to both the science of medical practice and the practitioner as the person who has to judge the evidence in relation to the patient. However, professional disciplinary action necessitates the externalization of that judgment when the codes are used to normalize the judgments of the professionals who have had complaints filed again them. The expertise of medicine acquires authority through its professional status in Canadian society, and the professional knowledge of good conduct gener-ates subject positions, or how physicians ought to self-regulate, how they ought to use evidence in the clinic. Colleges employ dis-cipline because, under liberal governance, they must continuously renegotiate trust with the public; the problematization of medical authority in the 1960s and 1970s is evidence of this (see Chapter 1).

Through the creation of standards such as CPGs and disciplin-ary procedures for self-governance the college shifts the "problem" of maintaining public trust to individual interactions in the clinic.

When it comes to professional competence, Liberal governance relies on technologies of the self. It is up to the physician to keep up to date on the best information, to constantly seek out the best practice, even if that means consulting CPGs. In her case study of the service industry in the United Kingdom, Fournier (1999, 293) found that "competencies operate through a combination of, on the one hand, standardization and codification of conduct ... and on the other hand, autonomisation of conduct." What this tells us about governing at a distance is that, when individual judgment is normalized through codes of conduct in order to discipline and to meet the objectives of governmental programs, the nature of the ethical substance of governmental programs is deresponsibilized. The art of self-governance is, thus, not only about self-development and being responsible so that one may act ethically but also about not judging the evidence at all.

Governmentality literature argues that governing is a "problematizing activity" (Rose and Miller 1992, 181). In Canada, liberal rule seeks to identify the problems of medicine, the predominant one being clinical judgment. Disciplinary programs "make the objects of government thinkable in such a way that their ills appear susceptible to diagnosis, prescription and cure by calculating and normalizing intervention" (183). Disciplinary rulings articulate what is desirable, the objective being that physicians have access to best practices to improve health care. And, given practical constraints on clinical activity, this means using CPGs. Solutions are to intervene in a way that is viable, that requires little investment from government, and that regulates individual activity at a distance. Osborne (1993, 345) describes the effects of these political rationalities as "inherently corrosive of the professions." The contradictory logic of liberal rule is that it produces more variation because regulation happens at the individual level, through the preservation of freedom of individual choices. The problematization of practice variation in medicine was to illuminate those choices in disciplinary decisions by individualizing the use of CPGs. In order for these strategies to be successful, the professionalization of governance necessarily deresponsibilizes judgments pertaining to these variations and problematized inconsistencies. Neoliberalism privileges "the advantages of regulation through local autonomy, it diminishes the scope for coherent [health care] service provision on the basis of a form of need determined by clinical truth" (354). The failure of EBM functions to allow government to "get away with" less health service provision because the problem with health care is conceptualized as the individual judgments made in the clinic and not as the access to resources (such as the time to review the literature) or improved health infrastructure (such as improved funding). Thus, better individual judgments are justified as the solution to better clinical care by the discourse of EBM itself.

Conclusion

THE HISTORY OF evidence-based medicine should not be thought about as a linear correction of the problems of clinical judgment. I do not explain the emergence of EBM as a quest for greater certainty regarding the effectiveness of clinical intervention, which led to the establishment of a new science of clinical epidemiology. And I do not explain the establishment of clinical practice guidelines either as a result of time constraints and the myriad sources of available evidence or as an innovation in clinical decision making. Instead, I attempt to persuade readers that the history of EBM should be thought about with respect to a social apparatus, a discursive and nondiscursive system that has been superimposed on the activities of the clinic. It is a system containing the following elements: production of a technique to normalize (i.e., CPGs) based on a "rationality" (the relations of discourse that delimit the science of clinical epidemiology), the disciplinary element of the medical colleges, the reintroduction of the perpetual problem of clinical judgment and the antithetical effect of deresponsibilization, and the repetition of the continuous reform of CPGs. It is the perpetuation of this system by liberal strategies of power that constitutes the dispositif of EBM.

The Impossible Clinic begins by considering the successes and crises of EBM. In order to understand these I trace the emergence of the concern with the use of evidence in clinical practice to the problematization of various aspects of clinical judgment in medical discourse after the Second World War. To put it in Deleuzian terms, by moving away from generality and focusing on the specificity of problems, I am able to render visible the nature of the problems to which statements and actions become solutions (cf. Deleuze 1994). By demonstrating that it was clinical judgment that was rendered visible as the target of thought and action – that is, the specific discursive practice that required intervention and amelioration – I analyze the relations of discourse and programs of conduct that are offered to resolve those problems as well as the solutions that are justified through the science of clinical epidemiology. If "evidence" is what physicians ought to use in order to make judgments, I explain how and under what social and historical conditions this concern emerged. The relationship between the laboratory sciences and the clinic, practice variation, medical authority, and other questions regarding systematizing clinical judgment are consistent with the main themes involved in problematizing it. That is, they illuminate and justify intervening in clinical judgment with new programs of conduct. As reform to medical education was one of the suggested resolutions to this issue, I engaged in a case study of the McMaster University medical program.

The relations of discourse that came to define clinical epidemiology were institutionalized at McMaster, the first department dedicated to this science in North America. The medical school program curriculum was influenced by the Department of Clinical Epidemiology and Biostatistics not only in the architecture of the social space of the teaching hospital but also in terms of training students to understand and use the information about the effectiveness of medical interventions by consulting and employing the methods of clinical epidemiology. Students would learn how to find, locate, and use this information in their practices. I show how the relations of discourse serve to justify the reorganization of human activity, and how, with the introduction of CE&B, clinical judgment could be assessed and surveilled. Further analysis of the McMaster medical school required me to spell out the effects of the program and the constitution of a particular kind of subject – the self-learner. Next, I examined the problem-based learning model, the emergence of its pedagogy and curriculum, and formulated the relations that responsibilized the self-learner: new graduates were responsible for keeping up with the literature, and they were trained to do so.

But how could the profession of medicine ensure that physicians were keeping up? For one thing, time constraints were a real barrier, and the problematization of practice variation continued to come up in the EBM discourse. It is here that I show how the convergence of EBM with the decision-making technology of CPGs enabled a particular strategy for intervening in clinical practice to become predominant. I demonstrate how CPGs resolved the ongoing problem of the up-to-date clinical judgment, and I expose the social conditions that allowed medicine to team up with government to create a national repository of guidelines in Canada. This relationship opened up new questions about the implementation of guidelines: What force, if any, did they have on clinical practice?

My question diverges from predominant questions in the sociology of medicine literature relating to evidence. I do not focus on how physicians understand or employ evidence or guidelines in their practices; rather, I explain the institutional mechanisms that regulate the use of guidelines and their effects. I focus on the provincial medical colleges in Canada. I construct a database of all disciplinary actions from 2010 until the time of writing to examine whether clinical judgments were normalized by CPGs in order to discipline those who made them. This database is the first of its kind to use Canadian data. I found that guidelines played a role in illuminating the difference between good and bad judgments in medicine. Complaints against physicians could be assessed by disciplinary committees on the basis of CPGs. Guidelines measured the difference between professional and non-professional conduct.

What are the effects of normalization on clinical judgment? What do these mechanisms act on? What do these mechanisms presuppose the nature of this substance to be? What must judgments be like so that disciplinary committees can use CPGs to successfully regulate (normalize and discipline) them? And, finally, what does this tell us about the role of professional governance? I use the term "deresponsibilization" to explain the effects of the convergence of these forces. When CPGs are employed to regulate, clinical judgment is conceived as externalized to the guidelines. The sanctions imposed on those who did not use CPGs in their practice indicate that CPGs are used to normalize professional judgments. The capacity of health practitioners to make judgments is targeted, which tells us that the improvement of population health is individualized to the clinic, and the physician's judgment is the target of biopower, which harnesses the physician's judgment in order to optimize it while simultaneously externalizing it. This finding reveals that EBM has failed because externalizing judgment to guidelines is antithetical to its goals, which are to teach new physicians to become lifelong learners, to learn to assess the evidence for themselves. These conclusions seem to confirm the worries of Greenhalgh and colleagues (2014) and those of even more recent philosophical critiques of medicine (e.g., Stegenga 2018). Despite this contradiction imposed on clinical judgment by the regulatory apparatus that governs medical practice, EBM goes on. So I attempt to explain why.

EBM continues despite its deficits because it is facilitated by liberal strategies of rule over and within the profession of medicine. Earlier I explain how the individualization of clinical judgment shifted focus away from system deficiencies and placed the onus of the improvement of health care on the doctors themselves rather than on government funding or infrastructure. What my conclusions offer to a sociology of medicine is a nuanced understanding of responsibility in professional regulation. I reveal how professional governance strategies that normalize individual judgments through general codes of conduct do not bring into being subject positions that recognize their personal responsibility to better themselves and their capacity to assess and judge the evidence. In fact, they can do the opposite, potentially having a deresponsibilizing effect on subjectivity and human activity. This is the heart of the contribution that *The Impossible Clinic* hopes to make to governmentality studies: the convergence of professionalization and normalization requires that sociologists rethink their understandings of subjectivity. As Rabinow and Rose (2006, 197) put it, governmental and biopolitical programs of conduct rely on "modes of subjectification" (i.e., subjects are "brought to work on themselves"); but this concept can be extended to include how subjectivity may not be *enlisted* but, rather, *externalized* when it becomes the target of professional strategies that deploy normalization to discipline members.

By specifying the nature of problems, sociologists can determine the limits of institutionalized ways of knowing and doing – specifically, the failures of institutional practices and the conditions that allow them to perpetuate. As a contribution to the institution of medicine, its clinical sciences and its professional sciences, I hope that *The Impossible Clinic* succeeds in historicizing that which appears to be dogma (or "given") in medicine's daily routines. I hope that I have clarified how the measures, principles, and practices that informed clinical practice at the bedside of medicine emerged, and how they responded to the main questions of the mid-twentieth century regarding clinical judgment. I serialize the problems that deal specifically with the clinic and the practices that seek to eliminate those problems not only as a response to the concerns of the times but also in relation to specific social and political contexts. In making a "family tree" of these questions, I describe the conditions of intelligibility that rendered certain discursive practices visible and the circumstances under which they emerged. I hope that I have illuminated the limitations of these programs of conduct. Not only are the effects of the strategies for intervention antithetical to the solutions, but the nature of this clinical problem can be neither resolved nor eliminated by the solutions so posed. For example, practice variation is an ongoing problem, and having better or more guidelines would not resolve it. EBM is not likely to be resolved as a result of this book, but I do hope that my genealogical work helps those in

the medical profession understand the mechanisms that are limit-
ing their ability to practice EBM and to improve health care more
generally.

Foucault and the Sociology of Medicine

Although it may seem undesirable to appropriate Foucault's
method for sociology, given his critique of the social sciences
(e.g., Foucault 1973b), through my commitment to a critical sociology I want *both* to explain the emergence of EBM and its failures *and* to update Foucault's work on the history of medicine.
Foucault's examination of the history of medicine was undertaken
during his archaeological period, when he focused on examining
medicine as a discursive formation. Further, chronologically, the
period of his investigations was mostly up to and including the
nineteenth century. According to Foucault's reflections, *Birth of
the Clinic* focuses its attention on locating and defining the combination of apparatuses that rendered medical knowledge "true."
Foucault's archaeology is concerned with how modern knowledge
is produced on two valences: 1) the discursive conditions that
give knowledge its truth character and 2) the specialized institutional settings in which experts can observe subjects and record
their activities. The operating theatre fulfilled both functions. It
was a physical space where physicians could make observations
and record the effects of disease on the human body. Knowledge
about the health of patients depended on the construction of
the theatre and the performance of autopsies. This became the
condition of seeing, of rendering disease visible, and of making
authoritative statements about the nature of the patient's problem (i.e., diagnosis). The conditions for the production of truth
depended on the reorganization of space in an institutional setting. This is much like the story of EBM and the "new" medical student, whose emergence depended on the construction of
a different kind of teaching hospital, one in which population
health research rendered individual clinical decisions visible
and in which the material organization of human activity gave

the applicability of epidemiological and biostatistical knowledge its authoritative character. Clinical judgments depended on the emerging visibility of decision making, whereby judgments about effectiveness acquired their truth character through a new science of population health, observation, and measurements of intervention and effectiveness at an aggregate level. My work extends Foucault's project by moving into the twentieth century, showing the institutional contexts within which clinical epidemiology could observe clinical decision making and the discursive preconditions of EBM, which is the dominant form of modern medicine: clinical judgments are considered true if they are evidence-based, and evidence is given its scientific character by clinical epidemiology.

My work also extends Foucault's by considering the effects of EBM and how they congealed through the convergence of institutionalized power relations. By widening the scope of my research to include the ways that the human sciences are used to target and intervene in human activity, which was one of the objectives of the genealogical method, I could shift my analysis to institutional relations and explain how knowledge about clinical judgment is put to work by regulatory programs to shape how individuals think about themselves and make themselves subjects of medical professionalism. Not only did the discourse of medicine problematize its practice in a way that determined what its problems were, it also shaped the kinds of solutions that became possible. Clinical judgments needed to be controlled, and so solutions that improved the capacity for clinicians to judge and control their decision making through normalization and professional discipline needed to be posed and implemented. Genealogical research reveals how the convergence of forces that channelled the production of knowledge (e.g., guidelines) came to influence emerging forms of subjectivity. EBM became dominant as a result of social conditions that mobilized the relations of discourse as a justification for the improvement of health care, which signals a biopolitical goal within liberal strategies of rule. Guidelines became dominant after they became evidence-based. Professional regulation mobilizes guidelines to render judgments visible so that they can be targeted for normalization – so that they can correct any deviation from what is considered best practice. Individual conduct can be regulated through questions about what to govern, about what kinds of knowledge justifies governmental intervention, and this occurs from a distance at the level of individual choices. My analysis extends Foucault's genealogical work by demonstrating that professional governance strategies are productive of certain kinds of subject positions: not necessarily "one who knows" but, rather, one who ought to recognize when to defer to the rules. These effects are antithetical to the goals of EBM; however, despite this fact, EBM continues because it allows for liberal programs of rule to relegate the responsibility of health care to individual decisions rather than to system-focused improvements in funding or infrastructure.

I hope that my work recommends genealogical analysis to the sociology of medicine as it allows sociologists to ask different kinds of research questions regarding how the human sciences shape how we understand institutions such as medicine, and how that shapes how we think about our health. By making links between the production of knowledge and the organization of human activity, sociologists and social scientists can investigate how institutions that seem "complete" today have actually become what they are and explain the effects they have on constituting subjectivity. Genealogical projects can go beyond merely describing relations of discourse. By showing how institutions have played a role in problematizing our existence – and in creating the systems of knowledge that constrain the kinds of questions that can be posed, the solutions that can be offered, and the programs that can be implemented – sociology can map the relationships between the human sciences and the power relations that mobilize and deploy them. Genealogy can explain the effects of such programs, their successes and their failures, and the social conditions that allow them to continue.

What the genealogical method brings to sociological analyses is its ability to shift our gaze away from the human/individual (or groups/collectives). Currently, questions in the sociology of medicine ask about how physicians use evidence or about the organizational barriers that inhibit the use of evidence or the production of evidence. These questions are important, but they do not offer a complete picture of how medical practice is organized within a social apparatus. As a major institution in a society that valorizes our vitality, invests in its maintenance, and regulates the production of knowledge about it, medicine is central to how we fashion our existence. Further to Foucault's (1973b, 357) point in *The Order of Things,* genealogical analyses can push beyond sociological projects that seek to locate conflicts that are produced as a result of our individual self-interests (e.g., physician resistance to CPGs) or contradictory group interests (e.g., medical power and the public).

The potential for future sociological research that chooses to embark on genealogical work relating to the evidence-based approach to medicine includes mapping the emergence of evidence-based practice in nursing and other health sciences as well as in complementary applied health sciences such as physio- and occupational therapy (e.g., Jewell 2011; Occupational Therapy Systematic Evaluation of Evidence 2019)[1] and alternative medicine (e.g., Kotsirilos, Vitetta, and Sali 2011). How does the EBM model operate in these practices? How has it become linked to or separated from its original conception? What were the institutional contexts in which this discourse could stabilize in other forms of practice? Understanding the proliferation of EBM in these related fields will provide further insight into the "lines of decent" in modern health sciences. I also think a great deal of additional research could shed light on the contingent relations that contribute to the perpetuation of EBM. I discuss the role of liberal governance as a deepening hierarchy between medicine and government. I leave aside the important relationships between EBM and economic constraints, EBM and commercialization, and EBM and the pharmaceutical industry (e.g., Matheson 2008; Abraham 2010). Future research on how EBM potentially benefits profit-seeking enterprises or fiscally conservative policies might also shed light on what allowed EBM to congeal in modern Western medical practice despite its failures. Sociology could play a major role in historicizing what has become common sense in clinical sciences across a variety of sites of practice. Additionally, actor network theory could build on my research by investigating the empirical impacts of CPGs and professional regulation by focusing on actual practices in the clinic.

Transformative Practices in Knowledge: Genealogy as a Counter-Human Science

Using Foucault's method has political implications over and above my contributions to a sociology of medicine informed by his genealogical approach.[2] Genealogical analysis helps to explain the connections between science and programs of conduct that seek to govern in particular ways in specific institutional contexts, but it can also provide the basis for "thinking otherwise" from within a dominant system of knowledge. Genealogy is a kind of critical socio-historical analysis: as a method, it explains the contingency of dominant modes of thought and action. I show what medicine "thinks" about clinical judgment, how it came to problematize its practice in a particular institutional setting. By showing that the problems of EBM are "political" insofar as they have a history and an objective (i.e., to intervene and improve health care), I explain how the effects of the forces that collectivize and individualize human activity in order to intervene and facilitate desirable outcomes acquire their authority on the basis of EBM. These analyses are beneficial: by illuminating the plurality of conversations that were once ongoing in the relations of discourse, and by showing how one particular set of questions became predominant, other, marginalized concerns can be examined and the conditions that led to their emergence can be questioned, explained, critiqued, and understood. Although the practices of medicine may be necessary and significant to society, the implications for the EBM program require analysis and reflection. By exploring the various lines of descent of our current world, alternative knowledge can be hypothesized, questioned, and considered, and the implications of any political strategy can be analyzed and critiqued. I conclude by discussing how genealogy allows sociology to formulate alternative knowledge and practices.

Genealogy can be considered a counter-human science. Like the theories of Marx, Durkheim, and Freud, genealogy shifts the gaze away from the individual (or groups of individuals) as the unit of analysis. All three of these social theorists explain that humans do not occupy centre-stage in our understanding of ourselves: we are imbricated in relations and institutions. Marx (1867) sought to explain modes of production in order to understand how social relations structure the state, including the revolution of technology and institutions like the family and religion. His intention was to explain the totality of relations in class-divided societies and their conditions of reproduction, not individual consciousness, which was merely a consequence of economic and social relations (cf. Marx 1859). Durkheim (1984) was interested in the study of social facts, not individuals. Social facts certainly influence individual consciousness in that they enable and constrain what we think and do, but they exist independently. Finally, Freud and Breuer (1952) demonstrated that the unconscious structures what we think and do without our being aware of it – it exists outside of our individual rationality. Freud and Breuer's science decentres the enlightenment project by showing that our motivations and experiences are not completely rational and that we are not always aware of them. There are desires and experiences that may be studied outside of our rational knowledge of them.

For Foucault (1973b, 378), the counter-human sciences are those social sciences, such as psychoanalysis and ethnology, that "are directed toward that which, outside man, makes it possible to know ... that which is given to or eludes his consciousness."

These social sciences examined objects that were not anthropological; rather, they focused, for example, on relations of historicity or the "unconscious" aspects of culture. For Foucault, such an approach, which can "do without a concept of man," does not mean a lack of scientific "rationality" or "objectivity"; it means that these sciences lead "back to their epistemological basis, and that they ceaselessly 'unmake' that very man who is creating and re-creating his positivity in the human sciences" (379). Appropriating this approach to the sociology of medicine opens up investigations into the kinds of things that become "problems" for society. Our investigations, however, would turn away from a "sociological explanation of phenomena manifested at the level of individuals" (380) and would turn, instead, toward the relations (i.e., discursive and strategic) that render such individualized problems knowable at particular points in time.

Social science could benefit from a *counter-human science* whereby we problematize institutions and social relations *not* individual or collective subjects. If it were to do so, the sociology of medicine, for example, would gain the ability to pose new questions about clinical judgment that, rather than individualize human interpretations or actions, ask how institutions came to restructure themselves on the basis of sciences that problematized the activities of human subjects. This approach shifts the gaze of sociology away from human subjects and toward institutions, to how they have changed, to the mechanisms that regulate them, and to the social relations that, over time, allow certain ways of knowing and acting to become dominant. It can also say something substantial about the regulatory effects of these relations. I expose the contradictions inherent to the liberal governance of clinical judgment, which is justified by the clinical sciences, as a failure of the goals of EBM. A benefit of my analysis is that it reveals that we do not need more or better educational programs, more guidelines, or better implementation at the professional level: these simply reproduce the problems that medicine aims to control. I hope that my work reveals that it is time to think otherwise, which requires looking beyond individual decision makers. Once the gaze is shifted, new projects can be executed and points of resistance can be located, which brings me to my final point about the role of genealogy and public scholarship.

Genealogy as Public Sociology

I have written about public sociology (Hanemaayer 2014; Hanemaayer 2018; Hanemaayer and Schneider 2014), which is a recent rebranding of a classic concern in the history of sociology: What is the relationship between sociology and social change? Can sociology engage and inform political projects? Genealogy positions the sociologist as what Foucault (1980b) refers to as the "specific intellectual." The public sociology debate was framed by Michael Burawoy (2005, 7), who describes public sociology as engaging with "thick, active, local publics" in order to "start a conversation" and to produce social change in the interest of "bettering humanity." According to him, this form of public intellectual comes in two forms: the "traditional" public sociologist and the "organic" (from Gramsci) public sociologist. The former engages with publics in unidirectional ways by generating research for wide audiences in the interest of educating them through the results of sociology, whereas the latter is more of an activist, located "on the ground" and working directly with the publics she "studies" to ameliorate their situations. Under the Burawoyan model, the plights of the publics with whom these forms of public intellectuals work is conceived in a humanist fashion. Genealogy can benefit those doing public sociology through its decentring move away from the individuals with whom the sociologist is imbricated.

Foucault's notion of the specific intellectual provides an alternative to Burawoy. The specific intellectual is not an individual who speaks for all. Foucault would be opposed to the idea that a sociology of medicine could speak *for* medicine about its history, its program or effects, or what its problems are or how to resolve them. *The Impossible Clinic* contributes to public sociology insofar as it analyzes the relationship between power and knowledge in evidence-based medicine. I highlight the contingent formation of clinical epidemiology, its measurements, and the social and political conditions that allowed it to stabilize across Western medicine; the role of medical colleges in creating and implementing clinical practice guidelines; the sanctions that effectively deresponsibilize; and the professional powers whose goal is to govern at a distance, thus constituting various subject positions in clinical practice. In doing so, I carry out a sociology of medicine that spotlights the weakness of governmental programs of conduct – programs that might otherwise seem "scientific." Evidence-based guidelines are antithetical to evidence-based medicine and, therefore, render it an impossible project.

By highlighting how the dispositif of EBM was able to continue due to liberal strategies of governance, I aim to function as a specific intellectual, who, according to Foucault, can direct attention to the weak points of institutions so that resistance and political projects can be undertaken. These political projects do not depend on individual humans doing things differently. In line with the commitments to a counter-human science, my contribution to a public sociology of medicine shows the contradictions that follow from evidence-based guidelines: they deresponsibilize, thus undermining the objectives of EBM. The advanced liberal logic that underpins professional governance strategies also produces greater variation, which was a problem EBM aimed to resolve. These are two weak points from which the institutional structure of medicine could be rethought. This would mean that change would not involve better implementation strategies or incentivizing the use of guidelines. Nor do the principles need to be revised (AGREE and GRADE have provided tools for ensuring that guidelines have the necessary rigour according to a clinical epidemiology hierarchy of evidence). However, the power relations that mobilize and deploy these scientific discourses can be resisted. Sociology can play a crucial role in disrupting knowledge-power relations, which means that we can begin to ask, in open public debate, what kind of medicine we want and what conditions would make its creation both viable and desirable.

Notes

Introduction

1 I am able to arrive at these conclusions because I take a different analytic approach to theorizing than do Timmermans and Berg (2003), who draw on a Weberian and Ritzerian analytic. For my part, I conduct a genealogical analysis that emphasizes force, contingency, and the discursive conditions of knowledge that organize the discursive and nondiscursive activities of the clinic. This approach allows humanities and social science scholars to grasp of the problems that generated the need to standardize, in the terms of Timmermans and Berg, and to explain how and why EBM has not achieved its goals. I take clinical judgment as the object of analysis, as the programmatic and problematic discursive practice of medicine, and I explain the conditions of its emergence as a result of the relations among various contingent forces.

2 For a discussion of genealogy as a method of effective history, see Dean (1994, 20): "Let us call history 'effective' to the extent that it upsets the colonisation of historical knowledge by the schemas of a transcendental and synthetic philosophy of history, and 'critical' in proportion to its capacity to engage in the tireless interrogation of what is held to be given, necessary, natural, and neutral."

3 Veridical statements concern questions about knowledge (e.g., what must be known?), whereas juridical statements concern the normative dimensions of intervention (e.g., what should be done?) (cf. Foucault 1979).

4 Certainly, important work has been done in this area. Consider, for example, Nikolas Rose (2007) on the molecularization of life. And there is also research on the use of new technologies and instruments to render the body visible in new and interesting ways (e.g., Fitsch 2011).

5 Paul Veyne (2008, 9) translates dispositif as "set up" to emphasize the assemblage of elements that is "set up" around a discourse.

Chapter 1: Conversations in Medicine

Acknowledgment: Chapter 1 and Chapter 2 feature material from Ariane Hanemaayer, "Evidence-Based Medicine: A Genealogy of the Dominant Science of Medical Education," *Journal of Medical Humanities,* 2016. Reprinted by permission from Springer.

1 For an excellent discussion of these topics, see Harry Marks's (1997) *The Progress of Experiment.*

2 Marks (1997), for example, documents various forms of resistance to the scientific model from within medicine.

3 Rheumatic fever is a condition that may develop in the heart after a group A Streptococcus bacterial infection, affecting the heart, joints, skin, or brain. While laboratory tests can determine whether or not the bacteria are present in the body, the diagnosis of rheumatic fever, at the time of Feinstein's writing, had no set objective procedure: it relied on a series of clinical criteria. Feinstein (1967) considered these criteria "subjective" as they relied on the clinician's interpretation of what they observed.

4 Each year since 1804, the Massachusetts Medical Society hosts an oration "to inform Massachusetts physicians of issues pertinent to current medical practice" (Massachusetts Medical Society 2013). Boardman's talk was titled "Dollars and Sense in Medical Care and Health Services: Relation."

5 For a history of the RCT see Bothwell and Podolsky (2016). The story of the success of the RCT is often attributed to the work of Austin Bradford Hill, a physician researcher working for the British Medical Research Council (MRC) in the 1940s who adapted the earlier scientific method of R.A. Fisher. Fisher's method, developed in the 1930s and 1940s, used population research to conduct trials on new therapeutic interventions. Hill, however, saw the effects of selection bias on the results of Fisher's work and, thus, added a randomization to the selection of patient participants (Chalmers 2003, 922).

6 I return to the Cochrane Collaboration in Chapter 2, where I discuss the social and political influences that enabled the proliferation of EBM.

7 See Knaapen 2013, 2014, and Teun Zuiderent-Jerak 2007 for similar concerns.

8 The study to which they are referring is McKibbon, Wilczynski, and Haynes (2004).

9 For details about the history and commercial success of tamoxifen, see Jordan (2003); for Viagra, see Irvine (2006).

Chapter 2: Institutional Sites

1 Letter from M.B. Dymond, Minister of Health, to Hon. John P. Robarts, Premier of Ontario, McMaster University Faculty of Health Sciences Archives [hereafter McMaster Archives], Series: Papers of J.R. Evans, 146.2, box 47, February 17, 1964.
2 McMaster had been petitioning the provincial government to be the location of a new medical program since the 1950s. In 1956, then president of McMaster University, G.P. Gilmour, wrote to Sir Francis R. Fraser, the director of the British Postgraduate Medical Federation, for advice on pursuing the formation of a second Ontario medical school at McMaster. Following the advice given to him in a letter sent in March 1956, President Gilmour wrote to the Ontario minister of education, W.J. Dunlop, to inquire about the possibility of choosing McMaster as a location for the formation of the medical school. He explained that there were a number of features that made McMaster an ideal location; for example, "a medical research laboratory [had] been maintained on the campus since 1948" (letter from President Gilmour to the Ontario Minister of Education, W.J. Dunlop, McMaster Archives, Series: Papers of J.R. Evans 146.2, box 47, March 1956, 5). Gilmour's successor, President H.G. Thode, continued to pursue the development of a medical school at McMaster. It was not until the annual 1962 meeting between McMaster University and the Ontario government's Committee on University Affairs that there was a written agreement stating that McMaster University in Hamilton "was the logical site for the next medical school" (Minutes, McMaster University and the Committee of University Affairs, Archives of Ontario [hereafter AO], RG 32-23, box 354145, 1963).
3 Report, "McMaster University and Medical Education," from Vice-President and Director of Research H.G. Thode to Premier Robarts, AO, RG 32-23, box B354145, January 13, 1961.
4 Report, "McMaster University for the Committee on University Affairs," AO, RG 32-54, box B177915, 1966, 1.
5 Memo, "Minister of University Affairs, for the information of the prime minister [i.e., premier] RE: Report of the Royal Commission on Health Services," AO, RG 32-54, box B177915, 1964, 1.
6 Dollar amounts in brackets have been converted to current (2019) Canadian dollars using the Bank of Canada's data.

7 Committee of University Affairs Issues Books, AO, RG 32-11, box B241011, 1964, 190.

8 This three-year timeline (1964 to 1967) proved to be too tight for the McMaster goal, and the first class was later pushed back to the fall of 1969. There were five years between the Ontario Ministry of Education's investment in the medical school and the enrolment of its first class.

9 John Evans on the history of McMaster's medical program, McMaster Archives, Series: Papers of J.R. Evans, 145.8, box 44, n.d., 2.

10 Ibid., 3.

11 John Evans on the objectives of medical schools, McMaster Archives, Series: Papers of J.R. Evans, 145.8, box 44, 1966, 1.

12 Minutes from selection committee meeting on epidemiology McMaster University, McMaster Archives, Series: Papers of J.F. Mustard, 151.5, box 33, December 7, 1967.

13 Department of CE&B Five-Year Overview 1986–91, McMaster Archives, Series: Clinical Epidemiology and Biostatistics, 184.5, box 001, 1991, 4.

14 Ibid.

15 Report on the Committee on University Affairs, AO, RG 32-23, B354530, 1968, 18.

16 In the following chapter, I discuss this approach and problem-based learning as well as its effects on the organization of medical activity.

17 Prospectus, McMaster Archives, Series: Papers of J.R. Evans, 144.6, box 33. n.d., 6.

18 Ibid., 7.

19 Objectives of the Department of Clinical Epidemiology and Biostatistics, McMaster Archives, Series: Clinical Epidemiology and Biostatistics, 184.5, box 001, 1972, 5.

20 Objectives of the Faculty of Medicine of McMaster University, McMaster Archives, Series: Clinical Epidemiology and Biostatistics, 184.5, box 001, 1969, 1.

21 Ibid., 2.

22 Ibid., 3.

23 Ibid., 4.

24 Ibid., 7.

25 Ibid.

26 Ibid., 9.

27 Educational Objectives in the Undergraduate Medical Curriculum, McMaster Archives, Series: Papers of J.R. Evans, 144.7, box 34, 1969, 1.

28 Objectives of the Faculty of Medicine of McMaster University, McMaster Archives, Series Clinical Epidemiology and Biostatistics, 184.5, box 001, 1969, 3.

29 Ibid., 11.

30 Revised Statement of General Goals – MD Program, McMaster Archives, Series: Papers of J.R. Evans, 145.8, box 44, 1972, 1.4(b), emphasis added.

31 Ontario Health Resources Development Fund for Capital Construction, AO, RG 32-23, B350860, 1969.

32 Ibid., 4.

33 Initially, twenty students enrolled in the first year of the McMaster medical program. These students were housed in temporary quarters while the complex was completed. The enrolment targets of sixty-four incoming students per year would be met once the proper facilities could be completed. The new facility would not open until 1971, two years after the first enrolled class, due to delays in labour and to union conflicts.

34 Health facilities, AO, RG 32-23, B356178, 1971, 34.

35 Objectives of the Faculty of Medicine of McMaster University, McMaster Archives, Series: Clinical Epidemiology and Biostatistics, 184.5, box 001, 1969, 9.

36 *Forum*, June Newsletter, AO, RG 32-23, B356178, 1971, 31–32.

37 Revised Statement of General Goals – MD Program, McMaster Archives, Series: Papers of J.R. Evans, 145.8, box 44, n.d., 6.

38 Ibid., 6–7.

39 Letter from John Evans to Dr. T. McKeown, McMaster Archives, Series: Papers of J.R. Evans, 146.2, box 47, August 28, 1967.

40 Letter from David Sackett to Mr. E.H. Zeidler, McMaster Archives, Series: Papers of J.R. Evans, 144.7, box 34, January 30, 1968.

41 Letter from David Sackett to G.P. Hiebert, McMaster Archives, Series: Papers of J.F. Mustard, 151.5, box 33, November 21, 1968.

42 Ontario Health Resources Development Fund for Capital Construction, AO, RG 32-23, B350860, 1969.

43 National Seminar on Health Care Evaluation, McMaster Archives, Series: Clinical Epidemiology and Biostatistics, 184.5, box 002, 1971.

44 Ibid.

45 Letter from H.H. Walker, Deputy Minister of Education, McMaster Archives, Series: Papers of J.R. Evans, 146.2, box 47, June 18, 1971.

46 Minutes, Committee on University Affairs, AO, RG 32-2, B167431, 1969, 4.

47 Department Overview, McMaster Archives, Series: Clinical Epidemiology and Biostatistics, 184.5, box 001, 1994, 51.

48 Report of First Annual Meeting of INCLEN, McMaster Archives, Series Education: Victor Neufeld, 215.6, box 003, 1983, 1.

49 Ibid., 4–5.

50 Annual report, July 1, 1980–June 30, 1982, McMaster Archives, Series: Papers of J.F. Mustard, 151.5, box 33, 1982.

51 A Course on Critical Appraisal of Data, McMaster Archives, Series Education: Victor Neufeld, 215.6, box 003, 1981, 2.

52 Department of CE&B Five-Year Overview 1986–1991. McMaster Archives, Series: Clinical Epidemiology and Biostatistics, 184.5, box 001, 1991.

53 Ibid., 5–6.

54 In *The Philosophy of Evidence-Based Medicine,* Jeremy Howick (2011) concludes that, with a few caveats, the methods of EBM do, in fact, provide valid knowledge on which clinical practice can be based (see chaps. 10 and 11).

55 Department Overview, McMaster Archives, Series: Clinical Epidemiology and Biostatistics, 184.5, box 001, 1994, 52.

56 Ibid., 3.

57 Ibid.

58 Ibid., 1.

59 CE&B Newsletter, McMaster Archives, Series: Clinical Epidemiology and Biostatistics, 184.5, box 001, 1992, 2.

60 Medical Research Council Response to the Rothschild Report, National Archives [hereafter NA] RG UGC 30/71, 1971.

61 Ibid., 3–4.

62 Research and Development Programme Budget Committee, 1978–79, NA, RG MH 148/1162, 1980.

63 In a phone conversation with the author in April, 2013, Sir Dr. Gray said: "At that time, the strategy was, get money and give it to Iain Chalmers." After the success of the Cochrane database and its commitments to *applied* research, these initiatives were well funded by government funds.

64 Department Overview, McMaster Archives, Series: Clinical Epidemiology and Biostatistics, 184.5, box 001, 1994, 1.

65 CE&B Newsletter, McMaster Archives, Series Clinical Epidemiology and Biostatistics, 184.5, box 001, 2000, 7.

66 Ibid., 2002, 18.

67 CE&B Newsletter, McMaster Archives, Series Clinical Epidemiology and Biostatistics, 184.5, box 001, 2002.

68 Ibid., 3.

Chapter 3: Responsibilizing a New Kind of Clinician

1 Objectives and Outline of the Undergraduate Educational Programme, McMaster Medical School, McMaster Archives, Series: Undergraduate Medical Education, 232.2D, box 001, April 1967, 1.

2 Minutes and Related Material, April–June 1969, McMaster Archives, Series: Undergraduate Medical Education, 232.1, box 020, May 1969, A2.

3 Objectives and Outline of the Undergraduate Educational Programme, McMaster Medical School, McMaster Archives, Series: Undergraduate Medical Education, 232.2D, box 001, April 1967, 1.

4 Ibid.

5 Ibid., 2.

6 Undergraduate Education Committee Curriculum Planning Outline, revised, McMaster Archives, Series: Undergraduate Medical Education, 232.1, box 020, May 1968, C1.

7 Ibid.

8 Ibid.

9 Ibid.

10 Ibid.

11 Students were exposed to computer technology early on to find "factual materials" when acquiring biomedical information. Undergraduate Education Committee Curriculum Planning Outline, Summer 1969, Phases I, II, McMaster Archives, Series: Undergraduate Medical Education, 232.1, box 020, 1969.

12 Ibid.

13 Minutes and related material, April–June 1971, McMaster Archives, Series: Undergraduate Medical Education, 232.6, box 003, May 12, 1971, 1.

14 Undergraduate Education Committee Curriculum Planning Outline, revised, McMaster Archives, Series: Undergraduate Medical Education, 232.1, box 020, May 1968, A1.

15 Ibid.

16 Ibid., E1.

17 Ibid., E2.

18 Undergraduate Education Committee Curriculum Planning Outline, Summer 1969, Phases I and II, McMaster Archives, Series: Undergraduate Medical Education, 232.1, box 020, May 1969, D2 (emphasis in original).

19 Undergraduate Education Committee Curriculum Planning Outline, revised, McMaster Archives, Series: Undergraduate Medical Education, 232.1, box 020, May 1968, E2.

20 Ibid., E3.

21 MD Undergraduate Education Program Goals and Objectives for Undergraduate Medical Education Final Draft, McMaster Archives, Series: Undergraduate Medical Education, 232.2, box 001, July 1971, I-3.

22 Undergraduate Education Committee Curriculum Planning Outline, revised, McMaster Archives, Series: Undergraduate Medical Education, 232.1, box 020, May 1968, E4.

23 Undergraduate Education Committee Curriculum Planning Outline, Summer 1969, Phases I and II, McMaster Archives, Series: Undergraduate Medical Education, 232.1, box 020, January 1969, 3.

24 Ibid.

25 Undergraduate Education Committee Curriculum Planning Outline, revised, McMaster Archives, Series: Undergraduate Medical Education, 232.1, box 020, May 1968, E5.

26 MD Undergraduate Education Program Review, McMaster Archives, Series: Undergraduate Medical Education, 232.2, box 001, November 1972, 23.

27 Ibid.

28 Ibid., 24.

29 Ibid., 25.

30 Undergraduate Education Committee Curriculum Planning Outline, revised, McMaster Archives, Series: Undergraduate Medical Education, 232.1, box 020, May 1968, F1.

31 MD Undergraduate Education Program Review, McMaster Archives, Series: Undergraduate Medical Education, 232.2, box 001, November 1972, 26.

32 Ibid.

33 Ibid.

34 Ibid., 27.

35 Undergraduate Education Committee Curriculum Planning Outline, revised, McMaster Archives, Series: Undergraduate Medical Education, 232.1, box 020, May 1968, G1.

36 MD Undergraduate Education Program Goals and Objectives for Undergraduate Medical Education Final Draft, McMaster Archives, Series: Undergraduate Medical Education, 232.2, box 001, July 1971, III-1.

37 Undergraduate Education Committee Curriculum Planning Outline, revised, McMaster Archives, Series: Undergraduate Medical Education, 232.1, box 020, May 1968, G3.

38 Ibid.

39 Ibid., G7.

40 MD Undergraduate Education Program Review, McMaster Archives, Series: Undergraduate Medical Education, 232.2, box 001, November 1972, 29.

41 Ibid.

42 Minutes and Related Material, January–March 1969, McMaster Archives, Series: Undergraduate Medical Education, 232.5, box 002, January 1969, 1.

43 MD Undergraduate Education Program Goals and Objectives for Undergraduate Medical Education Final Draft, McMaster Archives, Series: Undergraduate Medical Education, 232.2, box 001, July 1971, IV-1.

44 Minutes and Related Material, January–March 1969, McMaster Archives, Series: Undergraduate Medical Education, 232.5, box 002, January 1969, 1.

45 Ibid., I2.

46 Ibid.

47 Ibid.

48 MD Undergraduate Education Program Review, McMaster Archives, Series: Undergraduate Medical Education, 232.2, box 001, November 1972, 31.

49 Ibid.

50 Ibid., 32.

51 Undergraduate Education Committee Curriculum Planning Outline, revised, McMaster Archives, Series: Undergraduate Medical Education, 232.1, box 020, May 1968, H1.

52 Undergraduate Education Committee Curriculum Planning Outline, Summer 1969, "The Horizontal Program," McMaster Archives, Series: Undergraduate Medical Education, 232.1, box 020, 1969, 1.

53 Ibid.

54 Ibid., 4.

55 Ibid., 1.

56 Ibid., 2.

57 Ibid., G2.

58 Horizontal Program Planning Committee, Minutes and Related Materials, May–December 1968, McMaster Archives, Series: Undergraduate Medical Education, 232.9, box 012, September 1968, 5–6.

59 Ibid., 8.

60 Ibid., May 1968.

61 Ibid., 2.

62 Undergraduate Education Committee Curriculum Planning Outline, Summer 1969, "The Horizontal Program," McMaster Archives, Series: Undergraduate Medical Education, 232.1, box 020. 1969, G5.

63 Ibid., emphasis in original.

64 Ibid.

65 Ibid., G6.

66 Ibid.

67 Ibid., G8.

68 Ibid., G9.

69 MD Undergraduate Education Program Goals and Objectives for Undergraduate Medical Education, Final Draft, McMaster Archives, Series: Undergraduate Medical Education, 232.2, box 001, July 1971, I-1.

70 Undergraduate Education Committee Curriculum Planning Outline, Summer 1969, "The Horizontal Program," McMaster Archives, Series: Undergraduate Medical Education, 232.1, box 020, 1969, 3.

71 Ibid.

72 Review of the MD program, McMaster Archives, Series Undergraduate Medical Education, 232.2, box 001, July 1971, V-1.

73 Ibid., V-2.

74 Minutes and related material, October–December 1972, McMaster Archives, Series: Undergraduate Medical Education, 232.6, box 003, December 1972, 1.

75 Undergraduate Education Committee Curriculum Planning Outline, December 1968, Revised, McMaster Archives, Series: Undergraduate Medical Education, 232.1, box 020, 1968, 2.

76 Ibid.

77 Ibid., 4.

78 Minutes and related material, October–December 1971, McMaster Archives, Series: Undergraduate Medical Education, 232.6, box 003, December 1971, 1.

79 Ibid., 5.

80 Ibid., 6.

81 MD Undergraduate Education Program Review, McMaster Archives, Series: Undergraduate Medical Education, 232.2, box 001, November 1972, 33.

82 Ibid.

83 Undergraduate Education Committee Curriculum Planning Outline, Summer 1969, Phases I and II, McMaster Archives, Series: Undergraduate Medical Education, 232.1, box 020, January 1969, A1.

84 Objectives and Outline of the Undergraduate Educational Programme, McMaster Medical School, McMaster Archives, Series: Undergraduate Medical Education, 232.2D, box 001, April 1967, 1.

85 Ibid.

86 Ibid., March 1967, 2.

87 Review of the MD program, McMaster Archives, Series: Undergraduate Medical Education, 232.2, box 001, July 1971, 2.

88 Minutes and related material, October–December 1970, McMaster Archives, Series: Undergraduate Medical Education, 232.5, box 002, 1970.

89 Ibid., 2.

90 Ibid.

91 Objectives and Outline of the Undergraduate Educational Programme, McMaster Medical School, McMaster Archives, Series: Undergraduate Medical Education, 232.2D, box 001, April 1967, 2.

92 Minutes and related material, October–December 1970, McMaster Archives, Series: Undergraduate Medical Education, 232.5, box 002, 1970, 4.

93 Ibid.

94 Ibid., 5.

95 Ibid., 6.

96 Ibid.

97 Ibid., 1.

98 Ibid., 2.

99 Ibid.

100 Ibid. 3.

101 Ibid., 4.

102 Minutes and related material, April–June 1971, McMaster Archives, Series: Undergraduate Medical Education, 232.6, box 003, May 1971, 2.

103 Minutes and related material, January–March 1971, McMaster Archives, Series: Undergraduate Medical Education, 232.6, box 003, January 1971, 3.

104 Ibid., 3–4.

105 Minutes and related material, April–June 1971, McMaster Archives, Series: Undergraduate Medical Education, 232.6, box 003, May 1971, 2.

106 Ibid., 5–6.

107 Undergraduate Education Committee Curriculum Planning Outline, May 1968, revised, McMaster Archives, Series: Undergraduate Medical Education, McMaster Archives, 232.1, box 020, May 1968, L/II-1.

108 Ibid.

109 Minutes and related material, January–March 1971, McMaster Archives, Series: Undergraduate Medical Education, 232.6, box 003, January 1971, 3.

110 Minutes and related material, July–September 1969, McMaster Archives, Series: Undergraduate Medical Education, 232.5, box 002, July 1969, 14.
111 Minutes and related material, April–June 1971, McMaster Archives, Series: Undergraduate Medical Education, 232.6, box 003, April 21, 1971, 1.
112 Review of the MD program, McMaster Archives, Series: Undergraduate Medical Education, 232.2, box 001, April 1972.
113 In Canada, medical school programs are accredited by the Royal College of Physicians and Surgeons.
114 Minutes and related material, April–June 1971, McMaster Archives, Series: Undergraduate Medical Education, 232.6, box 003, May 1971, 2.
115 Ibid., 3.
116 Ibid., 4.
117 Ibid.
118 Ibid.
119 Ibid., 5.
120 Ibid.
121 Workshop on Maintenance of Competence, Royal College of Physicians and Surgeons Archives [RCPSA], Series: Booklets, November 1988, 3.
122 Ibid., 6.
123 Maintenance of Competence (MOCOMP) Pilot Program: An Information Guide for Specialists, RCPSA, Series: Booklets, 1991, February 1992, 1.
124 Ibid., 5.
125 Ibid.
126 Ibid., 6.
127 Proceedings of the Federation of Medical Licensing Authorities of Canada Workshop: Maintenance of Competence//Monitoring of Performance, RCPSA, Series: Records/documents, April 1994, 2.
128 Ibid., 1.
129 Ibid., 2.
130 Ibid., 1.
131 Ibid., 3.
132 Ibid.
133 Ibid., 5
134 Ibid., 8.
135 Ibid., 10
136 Ibid., 15.

137 McMaster University Faculty of Health Sciences Archives, Series: Undergraduate Medical Education, 232.6, box 003, 1972. Minutes and Related Material, January–March 1972.

Chapter 4: Technologies of Regulation

1 The ultimate criterion for ranking evidence in this system is the guideline's outcome *for a patient:* "Recommendations depend on evidence for several patient important outcomes and the quality of evidence for each of those outcomes" (Guyatt, Oxman, et al. 2008, 997). At the time of this writing, the CMA is using this system in its CPG database.

2 Clinical research in major medical journals includes a section for recommendations for physicians to apply in their practices. Additionally, there are multiple resources available to enable physicians to search out CPGs for use in their practice. I discuss one for the Canadian context in the next subsection.

3 Because Ontario is the most populated province, with many decisions, the publicly available statements only date as far back as 2012. Only 146 physicians are included in my sample of CPSO decisions.

4 See list of abbreviations for provincial college abbreviations.

5 Further research could explore these cases in greater detail and, nationally, monitor the use of guidelines when complaints of this nature are brought to the attention of the colleges and forwarded to disciplinary committees and tribunals that are tasked with regulating and evaluating the accused member.

6 Assessing this claim about "intent" goes beyond the scope of the current research question. Only a qualitative or ethnographic investigation with members of disciplinary committees would be able to shed light on these concerns. Presently, I am focused on whether guidelines have been institutionalized as an index for conduct, in order to understand the effects of normalization in disciplinary committee decisions.

7 This word is sometimes translated as "subjectification."

Chapter 5: The Impossible Clinic

1 This article has not yet been translated into English. My interpretation is based on my own translation.

2 See the work of Graham (2016) and Graham and colleagues (2012) for an ethnographically informed account of how the governance of health interventions often fails to build infrastructure during health care reform. These governance strategies typically benefit certain dominant groups.

Conclusion

1 Interestingly, this initiative is associated, in part, with McMaster University.
2 This section builds on the work of Ronjon Paul Datta, whose lectures I attended at the University of Alberta in 2013. All appropriations to my work are my own and so, too, are any omissions or errors in my reasoning.

References

Abraham, John. 2010. "Pharmaceuticalization of Society in Context: Theoretical, Empirical, and Health Dimensions." *Sociology* 44 (4): 603–22.

Agoritsas, Thomas, Anja Fog Heen, Linn Brandt, Pablo Alonso-Coello, Annette Kristiansen, Elie A. Akl, Ignaci Neumann, Kar A.O. Tikkinen, Trudy van der Weijden, Glyn Elwyn, Victor M. Montori, Gordon H. Guyatt, and Per Olav Vandvik. 2015. "Decision Aids That Really Promote Shared Decision Making: The Pace Quickens." *British Medical Journal* 350 (7624). DOI: 10.1136/bmj.g7624.

AGREE Collaboration. 2003. "Development and Validation of an International Appraisal Instrument for Assessing the Quality of Clinical Practice Guidelines: The AGREE Project." *Quality and Safety in Health Care* 12: 18–23.

Alam, Asim, Jason Klemensberg, Joshua Griesman, and Chaim M. Bell. 2011. "The Characteristics of Physicians Disciplined by Professional Colleges in Canada." *Open Medicine* 5 (4): E167–72.

American Medical Association. 2013. "About JAMA Evidence." http://jamaevidence.com/public/about_jamaEvidence.

Barrows, Harold S. 1983. "Problem-based, Self-directed Learning." *Journal of the American Medical Association* 250 (22): 3077–80.

–. 1986. "A Taxonomy of Problem-Based Learning Methods." *Medical Education* 20: 481–86.

–. 1996. "Problem-Based Learning in Medicine and Beyond: A Brief Overview." In *Problem-Based Learning in Higher Education*, edited by LuAnn Wilkerson and Wim H. Gijselaers, 3–12. San Francisco, CA: Jossey-Bass.

Barrows, Harold S., and R. Tamblyn. 1979. *Problem-Based Learning: An Approach to Medical Education*. New York: Springer.

Barry, Michael J., and Susan Edgman-Levitan. 2012. "Shared Decision-Making – The Pinnacle of Patient-Centred Care." *New England Journal of Medicine* 366 (9): 780–81.

Bennett, Kathryn J., David L. Sackett, R. Brian Haynes, Victor R. Neufeld, Peter Tugwell, and Robin Roberts. 1987. "Teaching Critical Appraisal of the Clinical Literature to Medical Students." *Journal of the American Medical Association* 257 (18): 2451–54.

Berg, Marc. 1995. "Turning a Practice into a Science: Reconceptualizing Postwar Medical Practice." *Social Studies of Science* 25 (3): 437–76.

Berkwits, Michael. 1998. "From Practice to Research: The Case for Criticism in an Age of Evidence." *Social Science and Medicine* 47 (10): 1539–45.

Bluhm, Robyn. 2009. "Evidence-Based Medicine and Patient Autonomy." *International Journal of Feminist Approaches to Bioethics* 2 (2): 134–51.

BMJ Publishing. 2013. "Why Read." Accessed November 18, 2013. http://ebm.bmj.com/site/about/whyread.xhtml.

–. 2014. "Why Do I Need Evidence-Based Medicine?" http://besthealth.bmj.com/x/static/514524/decision-support.html.

Boardman, Donnell W. 1974. "The Dollars and Sense of Medical Care and Health Services: Relation." *New England Journal of Medicine* 291 (10): 497–502.

Bothwell, Laura E., and Scott H. Podolsky. 2016. "The Emergence of the Randomized, Controlled Trial." *New England Journal of Medicine* 375 (6): 501–4.

Burawoy, Michael. 2005. "2004 Presidential Address: For Public Sociology." *American Sociological Review* 70 (1): 4–28.

Bursztajn, Harold, Richard I. Feinbloom, Robert M. Hamm, and Archie Brodsky. 1981. *Medical Choices, Medical Chances: How Patients, Families, and Physicians Can Cope with Uncertainty.* New York: Delacorte Press.

Canadian Health Services Research Foundation. 2006. "Myth: Medical Malpractice Lawsuits Plague Canada." Accessed on April 20, 2019. https://www.cfhi-fcass.ca/Migrated/PDF/myth21_e.pdf.

Canadian Medical Association (CMA). 2004. "CMA Code of Ethics." CMA Online. www.cma.ca.

–. 2007. "Handbook on Clinical Guidelines." Accessed on January 2, 2014. http://www.cma.ca/multimedia/CMA/Content_Images/CMA Infobase/EN/handbook.pdf.

–. 2011. *Canadian Clinical Practice Guidelines Summit: Toward a National Strategy.* Toronto: Canadian Medical Association.

Canadian Medical Protective Association. 2012. "Physician Professionalism – Is It Still Relevant?" Accessed on October 25, 2014. https://oplfrpd5.cmpa-acpm.ca/duties-and-responsibilities/-/asset_publisher/bFaUiyQGo69N/content/physician-professionalism-%E2%80%94-is-it-still-relevant-.

–. 2014. "Physicians and Research: Understanding the Legal, Ethical, and Professional Obligations." https://oplfrpd5.cmpa-acpm.ca/en/legal-and-

regulatory-proceedings/-/asset_publisher/a9unChEc2NP9/content/
physicians-and-research-understanding-the-legal-ethical-and-professional-
obligations.

Caplan, Robert A., Karen Posner, and Frederick W. Cheney. 1991. "Effect of Outcome on Physician Judgments of Appropriateness of Care." *Journal of the American Medical Association* 265 (15): 1957–60.

Cassels, Alan. 2015. *Cochrane Collaboration: Medicine's Best Kept Secret.* Victoria, BC: Agio Publishing House.

Chalmers, Iain. 1979. "The Search for Indices." *Lancet* 314 (8151): 1063–65.

–. 1984. "Confronting Cochrane's Challenge to Obstetrics." *Journal of Obstetrics and Gynaecology* 91: 721–23.

–. 2001."Comparing Like with Like: Some Historical Milestones in the Evolution of Methods to Create Unbiased Comparison Groups in Therapeutic Experiments." *International Journal of Epidemiology* 30: 1156–64.

–. 2003. "Fisher and Bradford Hill: Theory and Pragmatism?" *International Journal of Epidemiology* 32 (6): 922–24.

Chalmers, Iain, and Brian Haynes. 1994. "Reporting, Updating, and Correcting Systematic Reviews of the Effects of Health Care." *British Journal of Medicine* 309: 862–65.

Chalmers, Iain, Jini Hetherington, Malcolm Newdick, Lesley Mutch, Adrian Grant, Murray Enkin, Eleanor Enkin, and Kay Dickersin. 1986. "The Oxford Database of Perinatal Trials: Developing a Register of Published Reports of Controlled Trials." *Controlled Clinical Trials* 7 (4): 306–24.

Chalmers, Iain, Larry V. Hedges, and Harris Cooper. 2002. "A Brief History of Research Synthesis." *Evaluation & The Health Professions* 25 (1): 12–37.

Chalmers, Iain, Murray Enkin, and Marc J.N.C. Keirse. 1989. *Effective Care in Pregnancy and Childbirth.* Oxford: Oxford University Press.

–. 1993. "Preparing and Updating Systematic Reviews of Randomized Controlled Trials of Health Care." *Milbank Quarterly* 71 (3): 411–37.

Chalmers, Iain, and William A. Silverman. 1987. "Professional and Public Double Standards on Clinical Experimentation." *Controlled Clinical Trials* 8 (4): 388–91.

Civil Service Department. 1971. *A Framework for Government Research and Development.* Cmnd. 4814. London: HMSO.

Clinical Epidemiology and Biostatistics. 1981. "How to Read Clinical Journals: I. Why to Read Them and How to Start Reading Them Critically." *Canadian Medical Association Journal* 124: 555–59.

Cluzeau, F., and AGREE Collaboration. 2003. "Development and Validation of an International Appraisal Instrument for Assessing the Quality of Clinical Practice Guidelines: The AGREE Project." *Quality and Safety in Health Care* 12: 18–23.

Cochrane, Archibald L. 1972. *Effectiveness and Efficiency: Random Reflections on Health Services.* London: Nuffield Provincial Hospitals Trust.

–. 1979. *Medicines for the Year 2000.* London: Office of Health Economics.

Cochrane Collaboration, The. 2013. "Our History." Accessed on January 3, 2014. http://ukcc.cochrane.org/our-history.

College of Physicians and Surgeons of Alberta (CPSA). 2014. "Alberta Methadone Maintenance Treatment: Standards and Guidelines." http://www.cpsa.ca/standardspractice/alberta-mmt-standards-guidelines-dependence/.

College of Physicians and Surgeons of British Columbia (CPSBC). 2010a. "Nelken, Mayer. Richmond, BC." https://www.cpsbc.ca/files/disciplinary-actions/2010-05-17-Nelken.pdf.

–. 2010b. "Professional Standards and Guidelines." https://www.cpsbc.ca/files/pdf/PSG-Conflict-of-Interest.pdf.

–. 2013. "Standards and Guidelines." https://www.cpsbc.ca/for-physicians/standards-guidelines.

–. 2015. Brown, Roy Alan. Vancouver, BC." https://www.cpsbc.ca/files/disciplinary-actions/2015-11-20-Brown.pdf.

College of Physicians and Surgeons of Manitoba (CPSM). 2010. "Inquiry IC1246. Anthony Hlynka." http://cpsm.mb.ca/cjj39alckF30a/wp-content/uploads/20100225hlynkaIQ.pdf.

–. 2013. "Inquiry IC1595. Stephen John Coyle." http://cpsm.mb.ca/cjj39alckF30a/wp-content/uploads/20130813Coyle.pdf.

–. 2015. "Bylaw #11 Standards of Practice of Medicine." Accessed on January 27, 2016. http://cpsm.mb.ca/cjj39alckF30a/wp-content/uploads/ByLaws/By-law%2011.pdf.

College of Physicians and Surgeons of Newfoundland and Labrador (CPSNL). 2010. "An Orientation Guide for New Physicians." https://www.cpsnl.ca/Web/Files/cpsnl%20orientation%20guide%20rev%20April%202010(1).pdf.

College of Physicians and Surgeons of Nova Scotia (CPSNS). 2014. "Summary of Decision of Investigation Committee "c" for Dr. Philip Davis." Accessed on January 27, 2016. http://www.cpsns.ns.ca/Complaints-Investigations/Disciplinary-Decisions/Details/ArticleId/184/College-Issues-Consensual-Reprimand-of-Dr-Philip-Davis.

–. 2015. "Summary of Decision of Investigation Committee 'c' for Dr. Trevor Locke." http://www.cpsns.ns.ca/Portals/0/PDFcomplaints/Dr.%20Locke%20-%20Summary%20of%20Decision.pdf.

College of Physicians and Surgeons of Ontario (CPSO). 2007. "Practice Guide." http://www.cpso.on.ca/uploadedFiles/policies/guides/PracticeGuideExtract_08.pdf.

–. 2010. "Independent Health Facilities: Clinical Practice Parameters and Facility Standards – Sleep Medicine." http://www.cpso.on.ca/uploadedFiles/policies/guidelines/facilties/Sleep-Medicine-CPP-FS-2013.pdf.

–. 2011. "Methadone Maintenance Treatment Program Standards and Clinical Guidelines." http://www.cpso.on.ca/uploadedFiles/members/MMT-Guidelines.pdf.

–. 2012. "Van Dorsser, John Gerard CPSO# 23727." Accessed on August 22, 2016. http://www.cpso.on.ca/public-register/doctor-details.aspx?view=4&id=%2023727.

–. 2013. "Sleep Medicine Facilities." http://www.cpso.on.ca/uploaded-Files/policies/guidelines/facilties/Sleep-Medicine-CPP-FS-2013.pdf.

–. 2014a. "Haines, Alexander Milton CPSO# 59413." Accessed on August 22, 2016. http://www.cpso.on.ca/public-register/doctor-details.aspx?view=4&id=%2059413.

–. 2014b. "Reid, Robert Louis CPSO# 19827." Accessed on August 22, 2016. http://www.cpso.on.ca/public-register/doctor-details.aspx?view=4&id=%2019827.

–. 2015a. "Botros, Wagdy Adballa CPSO# 61884." Accessed on August 22, 2016. http://www.cpso.on.ca/public-register/doctor-details.aspx?view=4&id=%2061884.

–. 2015b. "Nicol, Olu-Kayode Louis Victor CPSO# 56525." Accessed on August 22, 2016. http://www.cpso.on.ca/public-register/doctor-details.aspx?view=4&id=%2056525.

–. 2015c. "Varenbut, Michael CPSO# 63881." Accessed on August 22, 2016. http://www.cpso.on.ca/public-register/doctor-details.aspx?view=4&id=%2063881.

Cooper, Melinda, and Catherine Waldby. 2014. *Clinical Labour: Tissue Donors and Research Subjects in the Bioeconomy.* Durham, NC: Duke University Press.

Cronje, Ruth, and Amanda Fullan. 2003. "Evidence-Based Medicine: Toward a New Definition of 'Rational' Medicine." *Health: An Interdisciplinary Journal for the Social Study of Health, Illness, and Medicine* 7 (3): 353–69.

Daly, Jeanne. 2005. *Evidence-Based Medicine and the Search for a Science of Clinical Care.* Berkeley, CA: University of California Press.

Datta, Ronjon Paul. 2007. "From Foucault's Genealogy to Aleatory Materialism: Realism, Nominalism, and Politics." In *Critical Realism and the Social Sciences: Heterodox Elaborations,* edited by Jon Frauley and Frank Pearce, 271–95. Toronto: University of Toronto Press.

Davidoff, Frank, Brian Haynes, Dave Sackett, and Richard Smith. 1995. "Evidence-Based Medicine." *British Medical Journal* 310: 1085.

Davis, A.J. 1981. "Medical Students' Concerns Must Be Discussed." *Canadian Medical Association Journal* 124 (May): 1194.

Davis, David A., Mary Ann Thomson, Andrew D. Oxman, and R. Brian Haynes. 1992. "Evidence for the Effectiveness of CME: A Review of 50 Randomized Controlled Trials." *Journal of the American Medical Association* 268 (9): 1111–17.

Dean, Mitchell. 1994. *Critical and Effective Histories: Foucault's Methods and Historical Sociology.* London: Routledge.

Deleuze, Gilles. 1992. "What Is a Dispositif?" In *Michel Foucault: Philosopher,* edited by Timothy Armstrong, 159–68. Hertfordshire, UK: Harvester Wheatsheaf.

–. 1994. *Difference and Repetition,* translated by Paul Patton. New York: Columbia University Press.

–. 1999. *Foucault,* translated by Seán Hand. London: Continuum.

Drachman, D.A. and C.W. Hart. 1973. "Complaint-Oriented Clinics." *JAMA* 20 (225): 996.

Durkheim, Emile. 1984. *The Division of Labour in Society,* translated by W.D. Halls. New York: The Free Press.

Easterbrook, Philippa. 1990. "'Critical Appraisal' or How to Interpret Journals." *British Journal of Medicine* 301: 392–93.

Eddy, David M. 1990a. "The Challenge." *Journal of the American Medical Association* 263 (2): 287–90.

–. 1990b. "Designing a Practice Policy: Standards, Guidelines, and Options." *Journal of the American Medical Association* 263 (22): 3077–84.

–. 1993. "Three Battles to Watch in the 1990s." *Journal of the American Medical Association* 270 (4): 520–26.

Elwyn, Glyn, and Adrian Edwards. 2009. "Evidence-Based Patient Choice?" In *Shared Decision-Making in Health Care,* 2nd ed., edited by Adrian Edwards and Elwyn Glyn, 3–18. Oxford, UK: Oxford University Press.

Engelhardt Jr., H. Tristram, Stuart F. Spicker, and Bernard Towers. 1977. *Clinical Judgment: A Critical Appraisal.* Dordrect, Holland: D. Reidel.

Erickson, Richard V., and Aaron Doyle. 2003. *Risk and Morality.* Toronto: University of Toronto Press.

Feinstein, Alvan R. 1967. *Clinical Judgment.* Baltimore, MD: Williams and Wilkins.

Feinstein, Alvan R., and Walter O. Spitzer. 1988. "The Journal of Clinical Epidemiology: Same Eine, New Label for the Journal of Chronic Diseases." *Journal of Clinical Epidemiology* 41 (1): 1–7.

Fitsch, Hannah. 2011. "(A)e(s)th(et)ics of Brain Imaging: Visibilities and Sayabilities in Functional Magnetic Resonance Imaging." *Neuroethics* DOI: 10.1007/s12152-011-9139-z.

Flanagin, Annette, and George D. Lundberg. 1990. "Clinical Decision Making: Promoting the Jump from Theory to Practice." *Journal of the American Medical Association* 263 (2): 279–80.

Fletcher, Robert H., Suzanne W. Fletcher, and Howard H. Wagner. 1982. *Clinical Epidemiology – The Essentials*. Baltimore, MD: Williams and Wilkins.

–. 1996. *Clinical Epidemiology: The Essentials*, 3rd ed. Baltimore, MD: Williams and Wilkins.

Foucault, Michel. 1972. *Archaeology of Knowledge*, translated by A.M. Sheridan. London: Tavistock Publications.

–. 1973a. *The Birth of the Clinic: An Archaeology of Medical Perception*. New York: Vintage Books.

–. 1973b. *The Order of Things*. New York: Vintage Books.

–. 1978. *History of Sexuality: An Introduction*, translated by Robert Hurley. New York: Vintage Books.

–. 1979. *Discipline and Punish*, translated by Alan Sheridan. New York: Vintage Books.

–. 1980a. "La poussière et le nuage." In *L'Impossible Prison, Recherches sur le système Pénitentiaire au XIXe siècle (L'Univers historique)*, edited by Michelle Perrot, 29–39. Paris: Seuil.

–. 1980b. *Power/Knowledge: Selected Interviews and Other Writings, 1972–1977*, edited by Colin Gordon. New York: Pantheon Books.

–. 1982. "The Subject and Power." In *Michel Foucault: Beyond Structuralism and Hermeneutics*, edited by H. Dreyfus and P. Rabinow, 208–26. Chicago: University of Chicago Press.

–. 1985. *The Use of Pleasure*, translated by Robert Hurley. New York: Vintage Books.

–. 1988. "On Problematization." *History of the Present* 4: 16–17.

–. 1989. *Foucault Live: Interviews, 1961–84*, edited by Sylvère Lotringer. New York: Semiotext(e).

–. 1991. *The Foucault Effect*, edited by Graham Burchell, Colin Gordon, and Peter Miller. Chicago: University of Chicago Press.

–. 1994. *Ethics: Subjectivity and Truth*, edited by Paul Rabinow. New York: The New Press.

–. 2000. *Michel Foucault: Power*, edited by James D. Faubion, translated by Robert Hurley. New York: The New Press.

–. 2003. *The Essential Foucault*, edited by Paul Rabinow and Nikolas Rose. New York: The New Press.

–. 2008. *The Birth of Biopolitics*, translated by Graham Burchell. New York: Palgrave Macmillan.

Fournier, Valérie. 1999. "The Appeal to 'Professionalism; as a Disciplinary Mechanism." *Sociological Review* 47 (2): 280–307.

Fowkes, F.G.R., and P.M. Fulton. 1991. "Critical Appraisal of Published Research: Introductory Guidelines." *British Journal of Medicine* 302: 1136–40.

Frauley, Jon. 2007. "Toward an Archaeological-Realist Foucauldian Analytics of Government." *British Journal of Criminology* 47 (4): 617–33.

Freud, Sigmund, and Joseph Breuer. 1952. *Studies in Hysteria*. London: Penguin Books.

Garland, David. 2001. *The Culture of Control: Crime and Social Order in Contemporary Society*. Chicago, IL: University of Chicago Press.

Godolphin, William. 2009. "Shared Decision-Making." *Healthcare Quarterly* 12: e186–e190.

Graham, Janice E. 2016. "Ambiguous Capture: Collaborative Capitalism and the Meningitis Vaccine Project." *Medical Anthropology: Cross-Cultural Studies in Health and Illness* 35 (5): 419–32.

Graham, Janice E., Alexander Borda-Rodriguez, Farah Huzair, and Emily Zinck. 2012. "Capacity for a Global Vaccine Safety System: The Perspective of National Regulatory Authorities." *Vaccine* 30 (33): 4953–59.

Greenhalgh, Trisha. 1999. "Narrative-Based Medicine in an Evidence-Based World." *British Medical Journal* 318, 7179: 323ff.

Greenhalgh, Trisha, Jeremy Howick, and Neal Maskery. 2014. "Evidence-Based Medicine: A Movement in Crisis?" *British Medical Journal* 348 (g3725). DOI: 10.1136/bmj.g3725.

Grimshaw, J.M., R.E. Thomas, G. MacLennan, C. Fraser, C.R. Ramsay, L. Vale, P. Whitty, M.P. Eccles, and L. Matowe. 2004. "Effectiveness and Efficiency of Guideline Dissemination and Implementation Strategies." *Health Technology Assessment* 8 (6): 1–94.

Grimshaw, Jeremy M., and Ian T. Russell. 1993. "Effect of Clinical Guidelines on Medical Practice: A Systematic Review of Rigorous Evaluations." *Lancet* 342: 1317–22.

Guyatt, Gordon. 1991. "Evidence-Based Medicine." *ACP Journal Club* 114: A16.

Guyatt, Gordon, Andrew D. Oxman, Gunn E. Vist, Regina Kunz, Yngve Falck-Ytter, and Holger J. Schünemann. 2008. "GRADE: What Is "Quality of Evidence" and Why Is It Important to Clinicians?" *British Medical Journal* 336: 995–98.

Guyatt, Gordon, and Drummond Rennie. 1993. "Users' Guides to the Medical Literature." *Journal of the American Medical Association* 270 (17): 2096–97.

Guyatt, Gordon, John Cairns, David Churchill, Deborah Cook, Brian Haynes, Jack Hirsh, Jan Irvine, Mark Levine, Mitchell Levine, Jim Nishikawa, and David Sackett. 1992. "Evidence-Based Medicine: A New Approach to Teaching the Practice of Medicine." *Journal of the American Medical Association* 268 (17): 2420–25.

Guyatt, Gordon, R. Brian Haynes, Roman Jaeschke, Maureen O. Meade, Mark Wilson, Victor Montori, and Scott Richardson. 2008. *Users' Guide to the Medical Literature,* 2nd ed., edited by Gordon Guyatt, Drummond Rennie, Maureen O. Meade, and Deborah J. Cook. Chicago, IL: McGraw-Hill.

Guyatt, Gordon, Sander J.O. Veldhuyzen van Zanten, David H. Feeny, and Donald L. Patrick. 1989. "Measuring Quality of Life in Clinical Trials: A Taxonomy and Review." *Canadian Medical Association Journal* 140: 1441–48.

Haas, Jack, and William Shaffir. 1982. "Ritual Evaluation of Competence: The Hidden Curriculum of Professionalisation in an Innovative Medical School Program." *Work and Occupations* 9 (2): 131–54.

Hanemaayer, Ariane. 2014. "Returning to the Classics: Looking to Weber and Durkheim to Resolve the Theoretical Inconsistencies of Public Sociology." In *The Public Sociology Debate: Ethics and Engagement,* edited by Ariane Hanemaayer and Christopher Schneider, 31–52. Vancouver: UBC Press.

–. 2018. "Genealogy as a Counter-Human Science." *Canadian Review of Sociology* 55 (2): 307–8. DOI: 10.1111/cars.12197.

Hanemaayer, Ariane, and Christopher J. Schneider. 2014. "Burawoy's Normative Vision of Sociology." In *The Public Sociology Debate: Ethics and Engagement,* edited by Ariane Hanemaayer and Christopher Schneider, 3–27. Vancouver: UBC Press.

Health Canada. 2003. "2003 First Ministers' Accord on Health Care Renewal." Accessed on January 3, 2014. http://www.hc-sc.gc.ca/hcs-sss/delivery-prestation/fptcollab/2003accord/index-eng.php.

–. 2004. "Royal Commission on Health Services, 1961 to 1964." Accessed on January 3, 2014.

Health Council of Canada. 2011. *Strategic Directions 2011.* Toronto: Health Council of Canada.

–. 2012. *Understanding Clinical Practice Guidelines: A Video Series Primer.* Toronto: Health Council of Canada.

Hill, Austin Bradford. 1948. "Streptomycin Treatment of Pulmonary Tuberculosis." *British Medical Journal* 2: 769–83.

Hunt, Alan. 1999. *Governing Morals: A Social History of Moral Regulation.* Cambridge, UK: Cambridge University Press.

–. 2003. "Risk and Moralization in Everyday Life." In *Risk and Morality,* edited by Richard V. Ericson and Aaron Doyle, 165–92. Toronto: University of Toronto Press.

–. 2004. "Getting Marx and Foucault into Bed Together!" *Journal of Law and Society* 31 (4): 592–609.

Howick, Jeremy. 2011. *The Philosophy of Evidence-Based Medicine.* Hoboken, NJ: Wiley-Blackwell.

Hurwitz, W. 2005. "The Challenge of Prescription Drug Misuse: A Review and Commentary." *Pain Medicine* 6 (2): 152–61.

International Clinical Epidemiology Network (INCLEN). 2013. "INCLEN." http://www.inclen.org/.

Irvine, Janice. 2006. "Selling Viagra." *Contexts* 5 (2): 39–44.

Jewell, Dianne V. 2011. *Guide to Evidence-Based Physical Therapist Practice,* 2nd ed. New York: Jones and Bartlett Learning.

Jordan, V. Craig. 2003. "Tamoxifen: A Most Unlikely Pioneering Medicine." *Nature Reviews* 2 (March 2003): 205–13.

Katz, N., R.C. Dart, E. Bailey, J. Trudeau, E. Osgood, and F. Paillard. 2011. "Tampering with Prescription Opioids: Nature and Extent of the Problem, Health Consequences, and Solutions." *American Journal of Drug and Alcohol Abuse* 37 (4): 205–17.

King, Lester S. 1983. "Medicine Seeks to be 'Scientific.'" *Journal of the American Medical Association* 249 (18): 2475–79.

Kleinman, Arthur. 1997. *Writing at the Margin: Discourse between Anthropology and Medicine.* Berkeley: University of California Press.

Knaapen, Loes. 2013. "European Regulation and Harmonization of Clinical Practice Guidelines." In *European Union Public Health Policy,* edited by Scott L. Greer and Paulette Kurzer, 64–80. London: Routledge.

–. 2014. "Evidence-Based Medicine or Cookbook Medicine? Addressing Concerns over the Standardization of Care." *Sociology Compass* 8 (6): 823–36.

Kotsirilos, Vicki, Luis Vitetta, and Avni Sali. 2011. *A Guide to Evidence-Based Integrative and Complementary Medicine.* London: Elsevier Health Sciences.

Lachlan, Farrow, Steve A. Wartman, and Dan W. Brock. 1988. "Science, Ethics, and the Making of Clinical Decisions: Implications for Risk Factor Intervention." *Journal of the American Medical Association* 259 (21): 3161–67.

Laine, Christine, and Frank Davidoff. 1996. "Patient-Centred Medicine: A Professional Evolution." *Journal of the American Medical Association* 275 (2): 152–56.

Lancet, The. 1995. "Evidence-Based Medicine, in Its Place." *Lancet* 346: 785.

Leplège, Alain, and Sonia Hunt. 1997. "The Problem of Quality of Life in Medicine." *Journal of the American Medical Association* 278 (1): 47–50.

Light, Donald Jr. 1979. "Uncertainty and Control in Professional Training." *Journal of Health and Social Behavior* 20: 310–22.

Matheson, Alastair. 2008. "Corporate Science and the Husbandry of Scientific and Medical Knowledge by the Pharmaceutical Industry." *BioSocieties* 3: 355–82.

Marks, Harry. 1997. *The Progress of Experiment: Science and Therapeutic Reform in the United States, 1900–1990.* New York: Cambridge University Press.

Marx, Karl. 1859. *A Contribution to the Critique of Political Economy*. Accessed on April 20, 2019. http://www.marxists.org/archive/marx/works/1859/critique-pol-economy/preface.htm.

–. 1867. *Capital*. Accessed on April 20, 2019. https://www.marxists.org/archive/marx/works/1867-c1/.

Massachusetts Medical Society. 2013. "MMS Annual Oration." http://www.massmed.org/About/MMS-Leadership/History/MMS-Annual-Oration/#.UecejZyAEmE.

McKibbon, Kathleen Ann, Nancy L. Wilczynski, and Robert Brian Haynes. 2004. "What Do Evidence-Based Secondary Journals Tell Us about the Publication of Clinically Important Articles in Primary Healthcare Journals?" *BMC Medicine* 2 (33). DOI: 10.1186/1741-7015-2-33.

McNamara, John J. 1972. "The Revolutionary Physician – Change Agent or Social Theorist." *New England Journal of Medicine* 287 (4): 171–75.

Medicine Act. 1991. Ontario Regulation 856/93: Professional Misconduct, S.O. 1991, c.30.

Merz, Beverly. 1983. "Medical Decision-Making: Analyzing Options in the Face of Uncertainty." *Journal of the American Medical Association* 249 (16): 2133–42.

Mulley, Albert G. 1988. "What Is Inappropriate Care?" *Journal of the American Medical Association* 260 (4): 540–41.

Mykhalovskiy, Eric. 2003. "Evidence-Based Medicine: Ambivalent Reading and the Clinical Recontextualization of Science." *Health: An International Journal for the Social Study of Health, Illness, and Medicine* 7 (3): 331–52.

Mykhalovskiy, Eric, and Lorna Weir. 2004. "The Problem of Evidence-Based Medicine: Directions for Social Science." *Social Science and Medicine* 59: 1059–69.

National Institute for Health and Care Excellence. 2013. "About NICE." http://www.nice.org.uk/aboutnice/.

National Opioid Use Guideline Group (NOUGG). 2010. "Canadian Guideline for Opioids for Chronic Non-Cancer Pain." http://nationalpaincentre.mcmaster.ca/opioid/.

Neville, Alan J. 2009. "Problem-Based Learning and Medical Education Forty Years On." *Medical Principles and Practice* 18: 1–9.

Norman, Geoff, and J.N. Blau. 1995. "Evidence-Based Medicine." *Lancet* 346 (8985): 1300.

Novas, Carlos. 2006. "The Political Economy of Hope: Patients' Organizations, Science and Biovalue." *BioSocieties* 1: 289–305.

Novas, Carlos, and Nikolas Rose. 2000. "Genetic Risk and the Birth of the Somatic Individual." *Economy and Society* 29 (4): 485–513.

Occupational Therapy Systematic Evaluation of Evidence. 2019. Accessed on April 17, 2019. http://www.otseeker.com/.

O'Malley, Pat. 1992. "Risk, Power and Crime Prevention." *Economy and Society* 21: 252–75.

Osborne, Thomas. 1992. "Medicine and Epistemology: Michel Foucault's archaeology of clinical reason." *History of the Human Sciences* 5 (2): 63–95.

–. 1993. "On Liberalism, Neo-Liberalism and the 'Liberal Profession' of Medicine." *Economy and Society* 22 (3): 345–56.

Osborne, Thomas, and Nikolas Rose. 1997. "In the Name of Society, or Three Theses on the History of Social Thought." *History of the Human Sciences* 10: 87–104.

Osborne, Thomas, Nikolas Rose, and Mike Savage. 2008. "Reinscribing British Sociology: Some Critical Reflections." *Sociological Review* 56 (4): 519–34.

Pease, Elizabeth. 1981. "Decisions." *Journal of the American Medical Association* 246 (15): 1731.

Rabinow, Paul, and Nikolas Rose. 2006. "Biopower Today." *BioSocieties* 1: 195–17.

Redelmeier, Donald A., and Eldar Shafir. 1995. "Medical Decision Making in Situations That Offer Multiple Alternatives." *Journal of the American Medical Association* 273 (2): 302–5.

Reiser, Stanley Joel. 1993. "The Era of the Patient: Using the Experience of Illness in Shaping the Missions of Health Care." *Journal of the American Medical Association* 269 (8): 1012–17.

Reveiz, Ludovic, Hernando G. Gaitán, and Luis Gabriel Cuervo. 2000. "Enemas during Labour." In *The Cochrane Library,* Issue 2, Update Software, Oxford, UK. https://doi.org/10.1002/14651858.CD000330.pub4.

Rose, Nikolas. 1993. "Government, Authority and Expertise in Advanced Liberalism." *Economy and Society* 22 (3): 283–99.

–. 2007. *The Politics of Life Itself.* Princeton, NJ: Princeton University Press.

Rose, Nikolas, Pat O'Malley, and Mariana Valverde. 2006. "Governmentality." *Annual Review of Law and Social Science* 2: 83–104.

Rose, Nikolas, and Peter Miller. 1992. "Political Power beyond the State: Problematics of Government." *British Journal of Sociology* 43 (2): 173–205.

Saarni, S.I., and H.A. Gylling. 2004. "Evidence Based Medicine Guidelines: A Solution to Rationing or Politics Disguised as Science?" *Journal of Medical Ethics* 30 (2): 171–75.

Sackett, David L. 1969. "Clinical Epidemiology." *Journal of American Epidemiology* 89 (2): 125–28.

Sackett, David L., and Marjorie S. Baskin. 1971. *Methods of Health Care Evaluation.* Hamilton, ON: McMaster University.

Sackett, David L., Brian Haynes, and Peter Tugwell. 1985. *Clinical Epidemiology: A Basic Science for Clinical Medicine*. Boston, MA: Little, Brown.

Sackett, David L., William M.C. Rosenberg, J.A. Muir Gray, R. Brian Haynes, and W. Scott Richardson. 1996. "Evidence-Based Medicine: What It Is and Isn't." *British Journal of Medicine* 312: 71–72.

Sackett, David L., Sharon E. Straus, W. Scott Richardson, and R. Brian Haynes. 2000. *Evidence-Based Medicine: How to Practice and Teach EBM*. Toronto: Churchill Livingstone.

Salwitz, James. 2012. "Against Medical Advice?" *Sunrise Rounds* Blog. http://sunriserounds.com/against-medical-advice/.

Satterfield, Jason M., Bonnie Spring, Ross C. Brownson, Edward J. Mullen, Robin P. Newhouse, Barbara B. Walker, and Evelyn P. Whitlock. 2009. "Toward a Transdisciplinary Model of Evidence-Based Practice." *Milbank Quarterly* 87 (2): 368–90.

Schechter, Alan N., and Robert L. Perlmanan. 2009. "Evidence-Based Medicine Again." *Perspectives in Biology and Medicine* 52 (2): 161–63.

Schoenbaum, Stephen C. 1993. "Toward Fewer Procedures and Better Outcomes." *Journal of the American Medical Association* 269 (6): 794–96.

Schmidt, H.G. 1983. "Problem-Based Learning: Rationale and Description." *Medical Education* 17: 11–16.

Schroeder, Steven A., Jane S. Zones, and Jonathan A. Showstack. 1989. "Academic Medicine as a Public Trust." *Journal of the American Medical Association* 262 (6): 803–12.

Silverstein, Marc D. 1988. "Prediction Instruments and Clinical Judgments in Critical Care." *Journal of the American Medical Association* 260 (12): 1758–59.

Smith, Dorothy E. 1990. *Texts, Facts, and Femininity: Exploring the Relations of Ruling*. New York: Routledge.

Smith, Richard, and Iain Chalmers. 2001. "Britain's Gift: A 'Medline' of Synthesised Evidence." *British Medical Journal* 323: 1437–38.

Starr, Mark, Iain Chalmers, Mike Clarke, and Andrew D. Oxman. 2009. "The Origins, Evolution, and Future of *The Cochrane Database of Systematic Reviews*." *International Journal of Technology Assessment in Health Care* 25 (S1): 182–95.

Stegenga, Jacob. 2018. *Medical Nihilism*. Oxford, UK: Oxford University Press.

Straus, Sharon E., and David L. Sackett. 1998. "Using Research Findings in Clinical Practice." *British Medical Journal* 317: 339.

Sudnow, David. 1967. "Dead On Arrival." *Society* 5 (1): 36–43.

Timmermans, Stefan, and Marc Berg. 2005. *The Gold Standard: The Challenge of Evidence-Based Medicine*. Philadelphia: Temple University Press.

Tosteson, Daniel C. 1990. "New Pathways in General Medical Education." *New England Journal of Medicine* 322: 234–38.

Vernon, David T.A., and Robert Blake. 1993. "Does Problem-Based Learning Work: A Meta-Analysis of Evaluative Research." *Academic Medicine* 68 (7): 550–63.

Veyne, Paul. 2008. *Foucault: His Thought, His Character.* Cambridge, UK: Polity Press.

Walters, William. 2012. *Governmentality: Critical Encounters.* New York: Routledge.

Waring, Justin. 2007. "Adaptive Regulation or Governmentality: Patient Safety and the Changing Regulation of Medicine." *Sociology of Health and Illness* 29 (2): 163–79.

Waugh, Douglas. 1984. "Medical Education: Challenges of the Future." *Canadian Medical Association Journal* 131: 145–46.

Weisz, George, Alberto Cambrosio, Peter Keating, Loes Knaapen, Thomas Schlich, and Virginie J. Tournay. 2007. "The Emergence of Clinical Practice Guidelines." *Milbank Quarterly* 85 (4): 691–727.

Wennberg, John, and Alan Gittelsohn. 1973. "Small Area Variations in Health Care Delivery." *Science* 182 (117): 1102–8.

Whelan, Emma, and Mark Asbridge. 2013. "The OxyContin Crisis: Problematisation and Responsibilisation Strategies in Addiction, Pain, and General Medicine Journals." *International Journal of Drug Policy* 24: 402–11.

White, Kerr L., Franklin Williams, and Bernard G. Greenberg. 1961. "Ecology of Medical Care." *New England Journal of Medicine* 265: 885–92.

White, Kerr L., P.B.S. Fowler, Fiona Bradley, Jenny Field, Neil Iggo, Geoffrey R. Norman, John Hughes, L.S. Chagla, P.G. McCulloch, Paul Aveyard, and David L. Sackett. 1995. "Evidence-Based Medicine." *Lancet* 346 (8978): 837–40.

Wulff, Henrik R. 1976. *Rational Diagnosis and Treatment.* Oxford, UK: Blackwell Scientific Publications.

Zuiderent-Jerak, Teun. 2007. "Preventing Implementation: Exploring Interventions with Standardization in Healthcare." *Science as Culture* 16: 311–29.

Index